Fast Facts

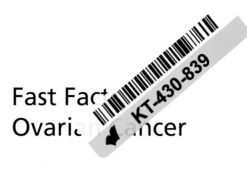

Fast Facts: Ovarian Cancer

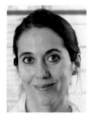

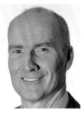

Christina Fotopoulou MD PhD
Consultant Gynaecological Oncologist
Queen Charlotte's and Chelsea Hospital
London, UK

Thomas J Herzog MD
Professor of Obstetrics and Gynecology
Deputy Director, University of Cincinnati Cancer Institute
The University of Cincinnati
Cincinnati
Ohio, USA

Declaration of Independence
This book is as balanced and as practical as we can make it.
Ideas for improvement are always welcome: feedback@fastfacts.com

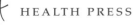

HEALTH PRESS

Fast Facts: Ovarian Cancer
First published May 2017

Health Press Limited, Elizabeth House, Queen Street, Abingdon,
Oxford OX14 3LN, UK
Tel: +44 (0)1235 523233

Book orders can be placed by telephone or via the website.
For regional distributors or to order via the website, please go to: fastfacts.com
For telephone orders, please call +44 (0)1752 202301

Fast Facts is a trademark of Health Press Limited.

A CIP record for this title is available from the British Library.

ISBN 978-1-910797-43-3

Fotopoulou C (Christina)
Fast Facts: Ovarian Cancer/
Christina Fotopoulou, Thomas J Herzog

Cover image: Three-quarters of ovarian cancer cases present at advanced stages
(III and IV) when the disease has already spread into the upper abdomen.
Intraperitoneal dissemination is the most characteristic feature of ovarian cancer.

Writing support for chapters 1, 2, 3, 4 and 8 from Michael Shaw PhD,
MScript Ltd, Hove, UK.
Medical illustrations by Graeme Chambers.
Typesetting by Thomas Bohm, User Design, Illustration and Typesetting, UK.
Printed in the UK with Xpedient Print.

List of abbreviations

AFP: alpha-fetoprotein

CA125: cancer antigen 125 (biomarker)

CT: computed tomography

CTLA-4: cytotoxic T-lymphocyte-associated protein 4

FGF: fibroblast growth factor

FIGO: International Federation of Gynecological Oncology

GCT: germ cell tumor

hCG: human chorionic gonadotropin

HE4: human epididymis secretory protein 4 (biomarker)

HGSC: high-grade serous carcinoma

HR: hazard ratio

HRD: homologous recombination deficiency

HRT: hormone replacement therapy

IP: intraperitoneal

IV: intravenous

MOGCT: malignant germ cell tumor arising in the ovary

MRI: magnetic resonance imaging

OS: overall survival

PARP: poly (ADP-ribose) polymerase (inhibitor)

PD-1: programmed cell death protein 1

PDGF: platelet-derived growth factor

PD-L1: programmed cell death ligand 1

PET: positron emission tomography

PFS: progression-free survival

PLD: pegylated liposomal doxorubicin

ROCA: risk of ovarian cancer algorithm

ROMA: risk of ovarian malignancy algorithm

SCST: sex cord–stromal tumor

STIC: serous tubal intraepithelial carcinoma

VEGF: vascular endothelial growth factor

WHO: World Health Organization

Introduction

In the last few years there has been a revolutionary increase in our knowledge of ovarian cancer management, from detection and genetics to surgery and novel targeted treatment approaches. This means that when it comes to detecting, diagnosing and treating women who have, or are suspected of having, ovarian cancer, there are significant opportunities for the well-informed healthcare professional to intervene in a meaningful way.

This resource offers a comprehensive overview of all levels of care, summarizing the most recent advances and putting them in a clinically meaningful context. It answers important questions such as when to operate and when to treat with various modalities, both conventional and novel.

We have striven to capture the key knowledge that a busy healthcare professional caring for patients with ovarian cancer needs, in a refreshingly readable concise format. After reading, please let us know at fastfacts.com if this resource has helped you to make better health decisions for your patients.

Epithelial ovarian cancer is the seventh most common cancer among women worldwide, with nearly 239 000 new cases reported in 2012.[1] It has the highest mortality of all gynecologic cancers, largely due to the fact that the majority of cases are not diagnosed until the disease has reached an advanced stage. Ovarian cancer often presents with a vague clinical picture, with gradual onset of non-specific symptoms that may be mistaken for those of other, benign, conditions such as the menopause or irritable bowel syndrome. A high index of suspicion is needed for prompt diagnosis, but even so, most cases will still present at advanced stages when the disease has already spread into the upper abdomen.

Incidence

The incidence of ovarian cancer varies markedly around the world: typically, the highest rates are seen in non-Hispanic white women, followed by Hispanic, African and Asian women (Figure 1.1).[1]

In the UK, there were 7378 new cases of ovarian cancer in 2014, accounting for 2% of all new cancer cases.[2] The age-standardized incidence rate in the UK is 23.3 per 100 000, which is the ninth highest in Europe, and it is anticipated that the incidence will increase by 15% between 2014 and 2035, reaching 32 per 100 000 women.[2]

In the USA, the age-standardized incidence of ovarian cancer is approximately 8.0 per 100 000 women, and the 1-year prevalence is approximately 11.8 per 100 000 (both the incidence and prevalence are higher in Canada, at 8.6 and 13.2 per 100 000, respectively).[3] Current US data suggest that 22 400 new cases will be diagnosed in 2017.[4]

Mortality

Ovarian cancer accounted for an estimated 152 000 deaths worldwide in 2012.[1] In the UK, approximately 4100 women died as a result of ovarian cancer in 2014, making it the fifth most common cause of

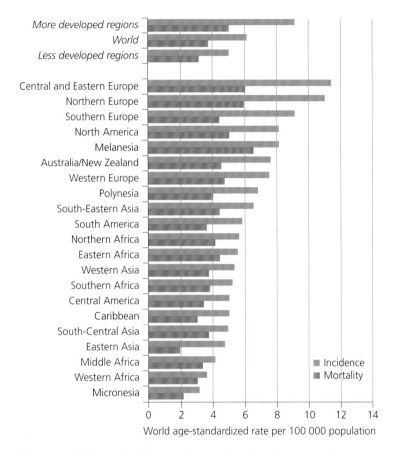

Figure 1.1 Estimated incidence and mortality of ovarian cancer by geographic region. Source: Ferlay J et al. GLOBOCAN 2012 v1.0. www.globocan.iarc.fr, last accessed 04 April 2017.[1]

cancer death among women.[2] Across the UK, the age-standardized mortality rate in 2014 was 12.9 per 100 000 population, with the highest rates in Northern Ireland and Wales (15.8 and 14.5 per 100 000, respectively) and the lowest in England (12.7 per 100 000).[2] In the USA, it is anticipated that ovarian cancer will account for approximately 14 080 deaths in 2017.[4] Mortality rates are disproportionately higher among women of African-American descent.[4]

Survival

Survival rates in ovarian cancer are the lowest of any gynecologic malignancy. Typically, 5-year survival rates are less than 50%, largely because three-quarters of cases are diagnosed at advanced stages (III/IV). Although age-standardized mortality rates are falling in many high-income countries, they are increasing in many low- and middle-income countries.[5]

Risk factors

Numerous factors have been reported to influence the risk of ovarian cancer (Table 1.1): age and genetic predisposition are among the most important factors associated with an increased risk, while oral contraceptive use, prolonged breast-feeding, tubal ligation and hysterectomy have been shown to be protective.

Age. The incidence of ovarian cancer begins to increase in women over 30–34 years of age, with the highest rates in women aged 65–69 years (Figure 1.2). In the UK, 53% of cases diagnosed between 2012 and 2014 were in women aged 65 years or older.[2]

TABLE 1.1

Confirmed and putative factors affecting ovarian cancer risk

Factors increasing risk	Factors reducing risk
• Increasing age	• Oral contraceptive use
• Genetic predisposition or family history	• Breast-feeding
• Nulliparity, infertility or celibacy	• Hysterectomy
• Early menarche, late menopause	• Tubal ligation
• Higher socioeconomic status	• Pregnancy
• Smoking	
• Exposure to asbestos	

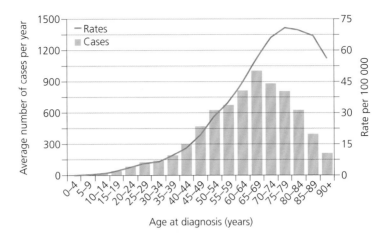

Figure 1.2 Incidence of ovarian cancer in the UK (2012–2014) according to age at diagnosis. Source: Cancer Research UK. www.cancerresearchuk.org/sites/default/files/cstream-node/cases_crude_ovary_I14.pdf, last accessed 27 March 2017.[2]

Genetics. The risk of ovarian cancer is approximately threefold higher in women with a first-degree relative (i.e. mother or sister) affected by ovarian cancer:[6] indeed, a positive family history is the strongest known risk factor for ovarian cancer,[7] even though 40% of patients with *BRCA1*- or *BRCA2*-related ovarian cancer have a negative family history.[8] Furthermore, as noted above, the incidence of ovarian cancer varies markedly between ethnic groups.[2] These findings clearly demonstrate the importance of genetic factors in ovarian cancer. However, the role of genetics is complex: specific genes have been implicated in both the development and progression of the disease, and in the response to therapy (Figure 1.3),[7] while the effect of individual genes may be modulated by environmental factors.[9]

Numerous genes have been implicated in the development of ovarian cancer (Table 1.2), of which the most common are *BRCA1* and *BRCA2* and the mismatch repair genes *MSH6*, *MSH2* and *MLH1*, which are also associated with colorectal and endometrial cancers. However, it is estimated that the genetic risk factors known at present account for less than half of the excess familial risk of ovarian cancer.[10]

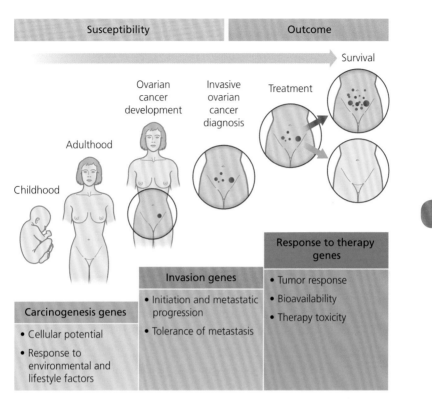

Figure 1.3 Potential genetic influences on ovarian cancer susceptibility and outcome. Adapted from Bolton KL et al. 2012.[7]

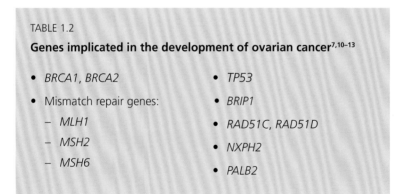

TABLE 1.2

Genes implicated in the development of ovarian cancer[7,10–13]

- *BRCA1, BRCA2*
- Mismatch repair genes:
  - *MLH1*
  - *MSH2*
  - *MSH6*

- *TP53*
- *BRIP1*
- *RAD51C, RAD51D*
- *NXPH2*
- *PALB2*

BRCA1 and BRCA2 are the strongest known genetic risk factors for ovarian cancer, accounting for around 65–85% of all cases of hereditary ovarian cancers.[13] The cumulative lifetime ovarian cancer risk associated with these genes is 40–50% for *BRCA1* and 20–30% for *BRCA2*.[7]

Mismatch repair genes. Inherited mutations in mismatch repair genes are associated with an estimated cumulative risk of ovarian cancer of 6–12%.[7] These genes account for 10–15% of hereditary ovarian cancers.[13] Mutations in these genes were first identified in patients with hereditary non-polyposis colon cancer (Lynch syndrome), who are also at increased risk of other solid tumors, including carcinomas of the endometrium, stomach, breast and pancreas.[13]

Other genes implicated in the pathogenesis of ovarian cancer include:
- the tumor suppressor gene *TP53*, which codes for a transcription factor involved in the control of cell proliferation and apoptosis[13]
- the double-strand DNA break repair genes *BRIP1*,[9] *RAD51C* and *RAD51D*[11]
- *NXPH2*, which encodes the signaling molecule neurexophilin 2.[12]

Reproductive factors. In general, factors that decrease the number of ovulatory cycles reduce the risk of ovarian cancer.[14]

Oral contraceptive use. In a landmark analysis of 45 epidemiological studies, the use of oral contraceptives was associated with proportional reductions in the risk of ovarian cancer of 15–29% over 5 years.[15] The protective effect of oral contraceptives increased with duration of use, and persisted for more than 30 years after discontinuation (Figure 1.4). On the basis of these results, the authors concluded that, at the date of publication (2008), oral contraceptives had prevented about 200 000 ovarian cancers, and 100 000 deaths from the disease and that the number of cancers prevented would rise to at least 30 000 per year over coming decades.[15] Similarly, a meta-analysis of six studies in women with *BRCA1* and *BRCA2* mutations showed that oral contraceptive use reduced the risk for ovarian cancer by more than 40% (odds ratio [OR] 0.58, 95% confidence interval [CI] 0.46–0.73) in this high-risk population.[16]

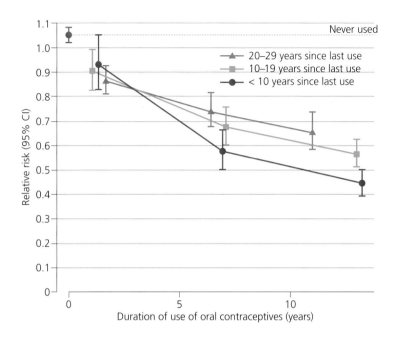

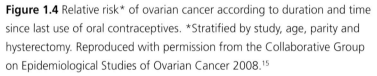

Figure 1.4 Relative risk* of ovarian cancer according to duration and time since last use of oral contraceptives. *Stratified by study, age, parity and hysterectomy. Reproduced with permission from the Collaborative Group on Epidemiological Studies of Ovarian Cancer 2008.[15]

Breast-feeding. Several recent systematic reviews and meta-analyses have shown that breast-feeding reduces the risk of ovarian cancer by 24–37%, and that the protective effect increases with the duration of breast-feeding.[17–19] The significance of breast-feeding as a protective factor was highlighted by a study in the UK, in which approximately 18% of cases were linked to women breast-feeding their children for less than 6 months.[20]

Hormone replacement therapy. Data from the Million Women Study showed that the risk of ovarian cancer was 53% higher in long-term (> 5 years) users of estrogen-only hormone replacement therapy (HRT) than in 'never users'. Similarly, the risk was 17% higher in long-term estrogen–progesterone HRT users than in never users.[21]

Environmental factors, including diet and obesity and exposure to talc, have been reported to influence the risk of ovarian cancer, but in many cases systematic reviews or meta-analyses have not demonstrated significant associations. One potential risk factor for which an association has been reported is smoking; in a meta-analysis of 51 epidemiological studies, including over 28 000 women with ovarian cancer, the relative risk (RR) of ovarian cancer was slightly but significantly increased in smokers compared with non-smokers (RR 1.06, 95% CI 1.1–1.11, p = 0.01).[22] Smoking was associated with an increased risk of mucinous cancers, but this was largely offset by a reduced risk of endometrioid cancers (see Chapter 2).

Prevention

Recognition of the importance of genetic and hormonal factors in the development of ovarian cancer has led to potential strategies for prevention of the disease. In particular, salpingo-oophorectomy is now widely recommended for high-risk (*BRCA1/2*-positive) women aged 40–45 years, once child-bearing is complete. A recent meta-analysis showed that prophylactic salpingo-oophorectomy reduced the risk of ovarian cancer by more than 80% (hazard ratio [HR] 0.19, 95% CI 0.13–0.27, p < 0.00001) in women with *BRCA1* or *BRCA2* mutations. It was also associated with a significant decrease in all-cause mortality (HR 0.32, 95% CI 0.27–0.38, p < 0.00001).[23] Iatrogenic menopause and its effects must be fully discussed with the patient.[23]

Screening

Despite the well-established genetic risk factors for ovarian cancer, no validated population-based screening programs exist. Close surveillance is recommended for women at high risk of the disease, especially those with *BRCA* mutations. Screening trials, as described below, have generally failed to demonstrate consistent effects on survival. The relatively low prevalence of the disease in the general population (1 in 70 lifetime risk), and the logistics of assessing small internal organs that may or may not have a long preinvasive or latent phase of cancer before spreading, probably contribute to the lack of an established screening strategy for ovarian cancer.

To date, the principal approaches to ovarian cancer screening have been the use of circulating biomarkers and ultrasound visualization of the ovaries. CA125 is the main biomarker in routine clinical use. Although it offers good sensitivity, levels of CA125 are low in the early stages of the disease and only increase in the later stages. Longitudinal measurements of CA125 using algorithms such as the Risk of Ovarian Cancer Algorithm (ROCA) offer greater sensitivity than single measurements with specified CA125 cut-off concentrations.[24]

Major trials of ovarian cancer screening

The UK Collaborative Trial of Ovarian Cancer Screening (UKCTOCS) evaluated 202 638 postmenopausal women who had annual CA125 measurements and transvaginal ultrasonography, ultrasonography alone or no screening at all.[25,26] After a median follow-up of 11.1 years, ovarian cancer had been diagnosed in 1282 women (0.6%). The primary analysis showed no significant reduction in mortality in the screened groups, compared with the unscreened group (Figure 1.5). However, a prespecified analysis that excluded prevalent cases showed a significant 20% reduction in deaths from ovarian cancer among women receiving multimodal screening: the overall reduction was 8% in years 0–7 and 28% in years 7–14.[26]

The UK Familial Ovarian Cancer Screening Study (UKFOCSS), a sister trial to the UKCTOCS, recruited 4531 women with an estimated lifetime risk of ovarian/fallopian tube cancer of at least 10%, based on family history or predisposing mutations.[27] The participating women underwent ROCA-based screening every 4 months. Transvaginal sonography (TVS) was performed annually if the ROCA results were normal, or within 2 months of an abnormal ROCA result. Risk-reducing salpingo-oophorectomy was encouraged throughout the study. Within a median follow-up period of 4.8 years, 4348 women underwent 13 728 women-years of screening.[28]

There was a significant shift toward earlier stages of the disease being detected within 1 year of screening: only 36.8% of the 19 cancers diagnosed within 1 year of screening were stage IIIb–IV compared with 94.4% of the 18 cancers diagnosed more than 1 year after screening ended (Figure 1.6).

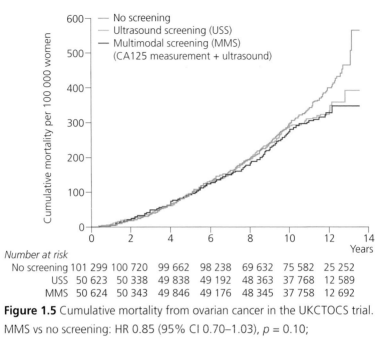

Number at risk

No screening	101 299	100 720	99 662	98 238	69 632	75 582	25 252
USS	50 623	50 338	49 838	49 192	48 363	37 768	12 589
MMS	50 624	50 343	49 846	49 176	48 345	37 758	12 692

Figure 1.5 Cumulative mortality from ovarian cancer in the UKCTOCS trial. MMS vs no screening: HR 0.85 (95% CI 0.70–1.03), p = 0.10; USS vs no screening: HR 0.89 (95% CI 0.73–1.07), p = 0.21. Reproduced from Jacobs IJ et al. 2016, under Creative Commons License.[26]

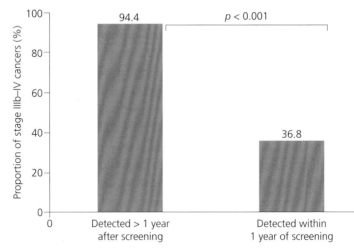

Figure 1.6. Proportion of advanced (stage IIIb–IV) ovarian or fallopian tube cancers detected in women according to the interval between screening and diagnosis.[28]

16

Screening also had a significant effect on the amount of postoperative residual disease and the degree of surgical complexity during cytoreduction: 94.8% of the 19 cancers diagnosed within 1 year of screening had no residual disease and lower surgical complexity, compared with 72.2% of the 18 cancers subsequently diagnosed.[28]

The study established ROCA-based screening as an option for women at high risk of ovarian cancer who defer or decline risk-reducing salpingo-oophorectomy, given its high sensitivity and significant stage shift. However, whether this strategy would improve survival in screened high-risk women has yet to be proven.

The US Prostate, Lung, Colorectal and Ovarian (PLCO) study included 78 216 women, aged 55–74 years, randomized to receive annual screening with CA125 for 6 years and transvaginal ultrasound for 4 years, or no screening.[29] Participants were followed for up to

---

Key points – epidemiology and prevention

- Ovarian cancer is the seventh most common cancer in women worldwide, and a leading cause of cancer death among women.
- The highest incidence rates are seen in non-Hispanic white women, and the lowest in African or Asian women.
- Survival rates in ovarian cancer are the lowest of any gynecologic malignancy, largely because the majority of cases are diagnosed at an advanced stage.
- Mutations in the *BRCA1* or *BRCA2* genes are the most important genetic factors contributing to an increased risk of ovarian cancer. However, the genetic risk factors known at present account for less than half of the excess risk of the disease.
- Oral contraceptive use is strongly protective against ovarian cancer.
- Risk-reducing surgery (salpingo-oophorectomy) is recommended for high-risk women up to the age of 45 years.
- To date, large screening trials based on CA125 measurement and transvaginal ultrasound have failed to show any significant benefits in terms of reducing deaths from ovarian cancer.

13 years. Screening had no significant effect on the incidence of deaths from ovarian cancer (RR 1.18, 95% CI 0.82–1.71), but surgery following false-positive diagnoses was associated with serious complications in 15% of patients. On the basis of these results, the US Preventative Services Task Force concluded that ovarian cancer screening should not be offered to women at low risk of the disease.[29]

References

1 Ferlay J, Soerjomataram I, Ervik M et al. *GLOBOCAN 2012 v1.0, Cancer Incidence and Mortality Worldwide: IARC CancerBase No. 11 [Internet].* Lyon, France: International Agency for Research on Cancer; 2013. www.globocan. iarc.fr, last accessed 04 April 2017.

2 Cancer Research UK. Ovarian cancer statistics. www. cancerresearchuk.org/health-professional/cancer-statistics/statistics-by-cancer-type/ovarian-cancer, last accessed 04 April 2017.

3 Global Cancer Observatory. www.gco.iarc.fr, last accessed 04 April 2017.

4 American Cancer Society. Cancer facts & figures 2017. www.cancer. org/research/cancer-facts-statistics/all-cancer-facts-figures/cancer-facts-figures-2017.html, last accessed 27 March 2017.

5 Webb PM, Jordan SJ. Epidemiology of epithelial ovarian cancer. *Best Pract Res Clin Obstet Gynaecol* 2016; October 3 [e-pub ahead of print].

6 Jervis S, Song H, Lee A et al. Ovarian cancer familial relative risks by tumor subtypes and by known ovarian cancer genetic susceptibility variants. *J Med Genet* 2014;51:108–13.

7 Bolton KL, Ganda C, Berchuck A et al. Role of common genetic variants in ovarian cancer susceptibility and outcome: progress to date from the Ovarian Cancer Association Consortium (OCAC). *J Intern Med* 2012;271:366–78.

8 Alsop K, Fereday S, Meldrum C et al. *BRCA* mutation frequency and patterns of treatment response in *BRCA* mutation-positive women with ovarian cancer: a report from the Australian Ovarian Cancer Study Group. *J Clin Oncol* 2012;30:2654–63.

9 Milne RL, Antoniou AC. Modifiers of breast and ovarian cancer risks for *BRCA1* and *BRCA2* mutation carriers. *Endocr Relat Cancer* 2016;23:T69–84.

10 Ramus SJ, Song H, Dicks E et al. Germline mutations in the *BRIP1, BARD1, PALB2,* and *NBN* genes in women with ovarian cancer. *J Natl Cancer Inst* 2015;107:pii:djv214.

11 Song H, Dicks E, Ramus SJ et al. Contribution of germline mutations in the *RAD51B, RAD51C*, and *RAD51D* genes to ovarian cancer in the population. *J Clin Oncol* 2015;33:2901–7.

12 Song H, Ramus SJ, Kjaer SK et al. Association between invasive ovarian cancer susceptibility and 11 best candidate SNPs from breast cancer genome-wide association study. *Hum Mol Genet* 2009;18:2297–304.

13 Toss A, Tomasello C, Razzaboni E et al. Hereditary ovarian cancer: not only *BRCA* 1 and 2 genes. *Biomed Res Int* 2015;2015:341723.

14 Kotsopoulos J, Lubinski J, Gronwald J et al. Factors influencing ovulation and the risk of ovarian cancer in *BRCA1* and *BRCA2* mutation carriers. *Int J Cancer* 2015;137:1136–46.

15 Collaborative Group on Epidemiological Studies of Ovarian Cancer; Beral V, Doll R, Hermon C et al. Ovarian cancer and oral contraceptives: collaborative reanalysis of data from 45 epidemiological studies including 23,257 women with ovarian cancer and 87,303 controls. *Lancet* 2008;371:303–14.

16 Moorman PG, Havrilesky LJ, Gierisch JM et al. Oral contraceptives and risk of ovarian cancer and breast cancer among high-risk women: a systematic review and meta-analysis. *J Clin Oncol* 2013;31:4188–98.

17 Luan NN, Wu QJ, Gong TT et al. Breastfeeding and ovarian cancer risk: a meta-analysis of epidemiologic studies. *Am J Clin Nutr* 2013;98:1020–31.

18 Li DP, Du C, Zhang ZM et al. Breastfeeding and ovarian cancer risk: a systematic review and meta-analysis of 40 epidemiological studies. *Asian Pac J Cancer Prev* 2014;15:4829–37.

19 Chowdhury R, Sinha B, Sankar MJ et al. Breastfeeding and maternal health outcomes: a systematic review and meta-analysis. *Acta Paediatr* 2015;104:96–113.

20 Parkin DM, Boyd L, Walker LC. The fraction of cancer attributable to lifestyle and environmental factors in the UK in 2010. *Br J Cancer* 2011;105(Suppl 2):S77–81.

21 Beral V, Million Women Study Collaborators, Bull D et al. Ovarian cancer and hormone replacement therapy in the Million Women Study. *Lancet* 2007;369:1703–10.

22 Collaborative Group on Epidemiological Studies of Ovarian Cancer, Beral V, Gaitskell K et al. Ovarian cancer and smoking: individual participant meta-analysis including 28,114 women with ovarian cancer from 51 epidemiological studies. *Lancet Oncol* 2012;13:946–56.

23 Marchetti C, De Felice F, Palaia I et al. Risk-reducing salpingo-oophorectomy: a meta-analysis on impact on ovarian cancer risk and all cause mortality in *BRCA 1* and *BRCA 2* mutation carriers. *BMC Women's Health* 2014;14:150.

24 Blyuss O, Gentry-Maharaj A, Fourkala EO et al. Serial patterns of ovarian cancer biomarkers in a prediagnosis longitudinal dataset. *Biomed Res Int* 2015;2015:681416.

25 Menon U, Gentry-Maharaj A, Hallett R et al. Sensitivity and specificity of multimodal and ultrasound screening for ovarian cancer, and stage distribution of detected cancers: results of the prevalence screen of the UK Collaborative Trial of Ovarian Cancer Screening (UKCTOCS). *Lancet Oncol* 2009;10:327–40.

26 Jacobs IJ, Menon U, Ryan A et al. Ovarian cancer screening and mortality in the UK Collaborative Trial of Ovarian Cancer Screening (UKCTOCS): a randomised controlled trial. *Lancet* 2016;387:945–56.

27 Rosenthal AN, Fraser L, Manchanda R et al. Results of annual screening in phase I of the United Kingdom Familial Ovarian Cancer Screening Study highlight the need for strict adherence to screening schedule. *J Clin Oncol* 2013;31: 49–57.

28 Rosenthal AN, Fraser LSM, Philpott S et al. Evidence of stage shift in women diagnosed with ovarian cancer during phase II of the United Kingdom Familial Ovarian Cancer Screening Study. *J Clin Oncol* 2017;35:1411–20.]

29 Buys SS, Partridge E, Black A et al. Effect of screening on ovarian cancer mortality: the Prostate, Lung, Colorectal and Ovarian (PLCO) Cancer Screening Randomized Controlled Trial. *JAMA* 2011;305:2295–303.

Further reading

Bowtell DD, Böhm S, Ahmed AA et al. Rethinking ovarian cancer II: reducing mortality from high-grade serous ovarian cancer. *Nat Rev Cancer* 2015;15:668–79.

Daly MB, Dresher CW, Yates MS et al. Salpingectomy as a means to reduce ovarian cancer risk. *Cancer Prev Res* 2015;8:342–8.

Dong A, Lu Y, Lu B. Genomic/epigenomic alterations in ovarian carcinoma: translational insight into clinical practice. *J Cancer* 2016;7:1441–51.

Doufekas K, Olaitan A. Clinical epidemiology of epithelial ovarian cancer in the UK. *Int J Womens Health* 2014;6:537–45.

Traditionally, it was believed that ovarian cancers usually originated in the surface epithelium of the ovaries. Although this theory supports the genesis of low-grade serous carcinoma, recent studies indicate that high-grade serous carcinoma (HGSC), the most common histological subtype of ovarian cancer, originates in the fimbria of the fallopian tubes (Figure 2.1).[1] Precancerous lesions, called serous tubal intraepithelial carcinomas (STICs) have been found on the fimbria in 5–10% of women with *BRCA1* or *BRCA2* mutations undergoing risk-reducing surgery and in up to 60% of unselected women with

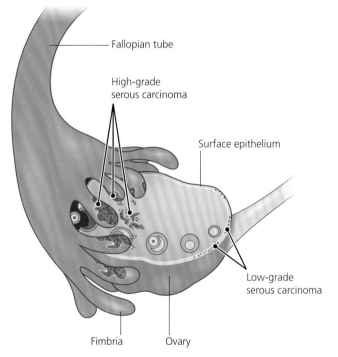

Fallopian tube

High-grade
serous carcinoma

Surface epithelium

Low-grade
serous carcinoma

Fimbria   Ovary

Figure 2.1. High-grade serous carcinoma has been shown to originate in the fimbria, a fringe of tissue around the ostium of the fallopian tubes, while low-grade serous carcinoma originates from the surface epithelium of the ovary.

pelvic HGSC. For this reason, the term 'ovarian cancer' should be considered a collective term that covers all ovarian–fallopial tube and primary peritoneal cancers.

Dissemination

Ovarian cancer cells tend to exfoliate into the peritoneum, where circulation of peritoneal fluid distributes them to the peritoneal surfaces and omentum. Indeed, intraperitoneal dissemination is the most characteristic feature of ovarian cancer; malignant cells can implant anywhere in the peritoneal cavity, particularly at sites of stasis within the peritoneal fluid circulation system.[2] The disease can spread via a number of mechanisms, including:

- local extension
- lymphatic invasion
- hematogenous dissemination
- transdiaphragmatic passage.[2]

Classification

The World Health Organization (WHO) histological classification of epithelial ovarian cancer is summarized in Figure 2.2. Epithelial tumors are the most common form of ovarian cancer, and the main focus of this book. The WHO classification for other forms of ovarian cancer are summarized in Table 2.1 and discussed in Chapter 9.

Epithelial tumors include benign, borderline and malignant histologies. Borderline tumors are a separate tumor entity characterized by complex papillary architecture, stratified epithelium with tufting (apparent detachment of cell clusters from their sites of origin), moderate nuclear abnormalities and moderately increased mitotic activity; in contrast to malignant tumors, they do not show stromal invasion.[3] The pathological characteristics of borderline tumors are:

- total microinvasive area < 10 mm^2
- depth of invasion ≤ 3 mm.

Epithelial cancers account for 80–90% of all malignant ovarian neoplasms,[4,5] of which HGSCs account for 70–74%, endometrioid tumors for 7–24% and clear cell carcinomas for 10–26% (Figure 2.3).

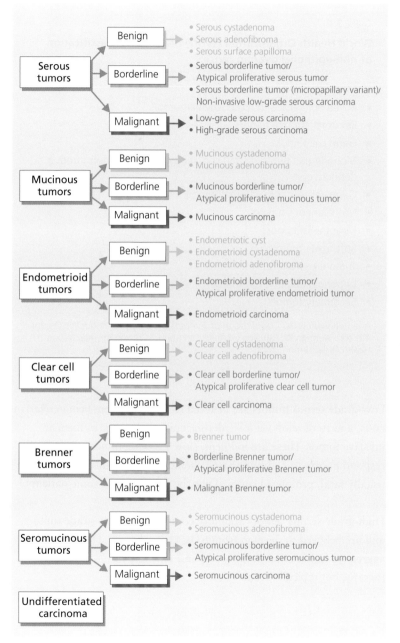

Figure 2.2. World Health Organization classification of epithelial tumors of the ovary.

TABLE 2.1

World Health Organization (WHO) histological classification of non-epithelial ovarian cancer

- Mesenchymal tumors
- Mixed epithelial and mesenchymal tumors
- Sex-cord–stromal tumors
- Germ cell tumors
- Monodermal teratoma and somatic-type tumors arising from a dermoid cyst
- Germ cell–sex cord–stromal tumors
- Miscellaneous tumors
- Mesothelial tumors
- Soft tissue tumors
- Tumor-like lesions
- Lymphoid and myeloid tumors
- Secondary tumors

Adapted from *WHO Classification of Tumours of Female Reproductive Organs*, 4th edn. Kurman RJ, Carcangiu ML, Herrington CS, Young RH, eds. World Health Organization, 2014.

Low-grade serous tumors are believed to originate from benign ovarian cysts, and to develop via a borderline epithelial tumor to form an invasive tumor. These are indolent, slow-growing tumors that usually respond poorly to platinum-based chemotherapy. Although they are usually fatal, prolonged survival may be achievable in some patients.[5]

High-grade serous tumors are more common than low-grade tumors, and are believed to develop from STICs (see above).[5] These are aggressive tumors that initially respond well to platinum-based therapy, but typically recur.[5]

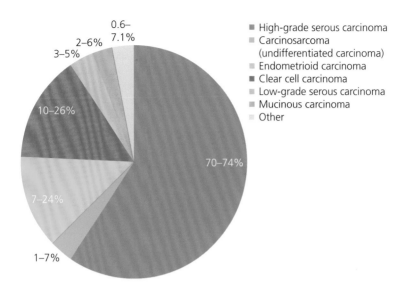

Figure 2.3 Proportion of epithelial ovarian cancers by subtype.
Source: *Ovarian cancers: evolving paradigms in research and care.*
National Academies of Science: National Academies Press, 2016. See also
Figure 2.2.

Key points – pathophysiology and classification

- Increasing evidence suggests that serous tubal intraepithelial
  carcinomas (STICs) in the fallopian tube are the most common
  precursor lesions of high-grade serous ovarian cancer, the most
  common type of epithelial ovarian cancer.
- Intraperitoneal dissemination is the most characteristic feature
  of ovarian cancer.
- Borderline ovarian tumors constitute a separate tumor entity
  and can present with the same histological subgroups as the
  invasive form of the disease.

References

1 Reade CJ, McVey RM, Tone AA et al. The fallopian tube as the origin of high grade serous ovarian cancer: review of a paradigm shift. *J Obstet Gynaecol Can* 2014;36:133–40.

2 Green A. Ovarian cancer. emedicine.medscape.com/article/255771, last accessed 04 April 2017.

3 du Bois A, Ewald-Riegler N, de Gregorio N et al. Borderline tumours of the ovary: a cohort study of the Arbeitsgmeinschaft Gynäkologische Onkologie (AGO) Study Group. *Eur J Cancer* 2013;49:1905–14.

4 Cancer Research UK. Ovarian cancer incidence morphology. www.cancerresearchuk.org/health-professional/cancer-statistics/statistics-by-cancer-type/ovarian-cancer/incidence#heading-Four, last accessed 04 April 2017.

5 McCluggage WG. My approach to and thoughts on the typing of ovarian carcinomas. *J Clin Pathol* 2008;61:152–63.

Further reading

National Academies of Science, Engineering, and Medicine. *Ovarian Cancers: Evolving Paradigms in Research and Care.* National Academies Press, 2016. www.nap.edu/21841, last accessed 04 April 2017.

As described in Chapter 1, genetic factors are an important determinant of ovarian cancer risk. Indeed, inherited genetic mutations are associated with about 15% of ovarian cancers, depending on the cancer subtype.[1] Furthermore, some epithelial ovarian cancers result from somatic mutations, as well as mutations in other genes that are critical in DNA repair pathways. Importantly, the absence of a family history of ovarian cancer may not preclude a genetic predisposition: inherited mutations may be present in up to 25% of women with high-grade serous carcinoma (HGSC), but up to half of these women may not have a family history of ovarian or breast cancer.[2,3] For these reasons, genetic testing has a valuable role to play in identifying women at risk of ovarian cancer.

It is important to differentiate between genetic counseling and genetic testing. Most experts stress that informed counseling should be given before genetic testing by a qualified healthcare professional, but not necessarily a genetic counselor. Currently, there is a shortage of counselors to provide timely consultations; hence, some propose direct genetic testing without counseling, with the reflex use of counselors for patients with positive or questionable findings.

The development of multiplex gene panel testing to sequence multiple genes simultaneously may identify more individuals with cancer gene mutations than *BRCA1* or *BRCA2* testing alone. This development, alongside a marked decrease in the cost of genetic testing,[1] means that routine genetic testing is now much more accessible than was previously the case.

Guidelines for genetic testing

A number of organizations have published recommendations and guidelines for genetic counseling and testing (also see Further reading, page 31).[4–6,8] Most of these recommend that all women diagnosed with epithelial ovarian cancer should undergo genetic testing, irrespective of their family history or age at diagnosis. The majority of guidelines

27

recommend that genetic testing should include both pre- and post-test counseling with a genetic counselor or other appropriate healthcare professional with expertise in cancer genetics.[1] The benefits of genetic testing in patients with ovarian cancer include:

- prognostic information for counseling
- predictive information that guides treatment with DNA-damaging agents such as poly (ADP-ribose) polymerase (PARP) inhibitors
- enabling amendments to screening recommendations and patient counseling, including consideration of surgical or non-surgical risk reduction strategies
- the opportunity for cascade testing of relatives (see below).

Cascade testing

Cascade testing is the testing of close blood relatives of individuals known to be at high risk of genetic conditions. If a genetic mutation (e.g. a *BRCA1* mutation) is identified through initial genetic testing of the patient, further testing for this mutation can then be offered to close blood relatives of the affected individual (Figure 3.1). Using this strategy, it is only necessary to test for the specific mutation, rather than performing multigene testing; as a result, the cost of testing can be significantly reduced.[1,7]

The problem of under-referral

Despite the potential benefits of genetic testing in terms of identifying women at high risk of ovarian cancer, referral rates for genetic counseling services are low. In one study, only 14.5% of women with ovarian cancer who should have been referred according to the US National Comprehensive Cancer Network guidelines received a referral for genetic counseling, and of those only 59.5% opted for counseling (although it should be noted that about 95% of women who received counseling subsequently underwent genetic testing).[8] Significant predictors for referral included:

- younger age
- diagnosis of breast cancer
- family history, and increasing number of affected family members
- earlier disease stage.[8]

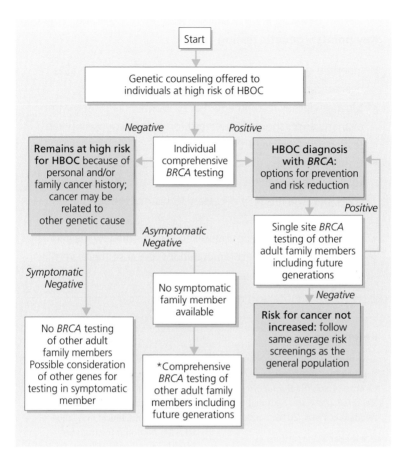

Figure 3.1 Cascade testing for *BRCA1* mutations for hereditary breast or ovarian cancer (HBOC). *Asymptomatic family members who wish to be tested will need comprehensive *BRCA* testing until a positive mutation is identified or a symptomatic family member becomes available for testing. Symptomatic is defined as being diagnosed with a hereditary breast or ovarian (HBOC)-related cancer. Adapted from George R et al. 2015.[7]

Low referral rates have also been reported in the UK. Studies have suggested that this may be partly because of a reluctance among primary care providers to assume responsibility for controlling access to specialized genetic services.[5]

Key points – genetic testing

- Inherited genetic mutations are associated with about 15% of ovarian cancers, depending on the histological subtype.
- Most guidelines recommend that all women diagnosed with ovarian cancer should be referred for genetic counseling and testing, irrespective of their family history.
- Cascade screening of close blood relatives of individuals found to carry specific genetic mutations can markedly reduce testing costs, because it is only necessary to test for the specific mutation.
- Referral rates to genetic counseling services are low, despite numerous guideline recommendations, because there are still significant funding issues.

References

1 National Academies of Science, Engineering, and Medicine. Ovarian Cancers: *Evolving Paradigms in Research and Care*. National Academies Press, 2016.

2 Schrader KA, Hurlburt J, Kalloger SE et al. Germline *BRCA1* and *BRCA2* mutations in ovarian cancer: utility of a histology-based referral strategy. *Obstet Gynecol* 2012;120:235–40.

3 Walsh T, Casadei S, Lee MK et al. Mutations in 12 genes for inherited ovarian, fallopian tube, and peritoneal carcinoma identified by massively parallel sequencing. *Proc Natl Acad Sci U S A* 2011;108:18032–7.

4 NICE. Familial breast cancer: classification, care and managing breast cancer and related risks in people with a family history of breast cancer. Clinical Guideline CG164. National Institute for Health and Care Excellence, 25 June 2013. www.nice.org.uk/guidance/cg164, last accessed 04 April 2017.

5 SIGN. Epithelial ovarian cancer. Section 2: screening and the role of prophylactic oophorectomy. Scottish Intercollegiate Guidelines Network, 27 August 2015. www.sign.ac.uk/guidelines/fulltext/75/section2.html, last accessed 04 April 2017.

6 Balmaña J, Diez O, Rubio I, Castiglione M; ESMO Guidelines Working Group. BRCA in breast cancer: ESMO Clinical Practice Guidelines. *Ann Oncol* 2010;21(Suppl 5):v20–2.

7 George R, Kovak K, Cox SL. Aligning policy to promote cascade genetic screening for prevention and early diagnosis of heritable diseases. *J Genet Couns* 2015;24:388–99.

8 Febbraro T, Robison K, Wilbur JS et al. Adherence patterns to National Comprehensive Cancer Network (NCCN) guidelines for referral to cancer genetic professionals. *Gynecol Oncol* 2015;138:109–14.

Further reading

Hampel H, Bennett RL, Buchanan A et al. A practice guideline from the American College of Medical Genetics and Genomics and the National Society of Genetic Counselors: referral indications for cancer predisposition assessment. *Genet Med* 2014;17:70–87.

Lambert M. ACOG guidelines for managing hereditary breast and ovarian cancer syndrome. *Am Fam Physician* 2009;80:1505–7.

Schorge JO, Modesitt SC, Coleman RL, Herzog TJ. SGO White Paper on ovarian cancer: etiology, screening and surveillance. *Gyn Oncol* 2010;119:7–17.

US Preventive Services Task Force. Risk assessment, genetic counseling, and genetic testing for BRCA-related cancer in women: recommendation statement. *Am Fam Physician* 2015;91:online. www.aafp.org/afp/2015/0115/od1.html, last accessed 26 April 2017.

Vergote I, Banerjee S, Gerdes AM et al. Current perspectives on recommendations for BRCA genetic testing in ovarian cancer patients. *Eur J Cancer* 2016;69:127–34.

Diagnosis

As outlined in Chapter 1, the majority of women with ovarian cancer (> 80%) are not diagnosed until the disease has reached an advanced stage. The initial diagnostic pathway of epithelial ovarian cancer is based on the assessment of symptoms and overall clinical picture, biomarkers (particularly CA125), family history and imaging.

Symptoms. Although ovarian cancer has previously been considered a 'silent killer', it is now recognized that a high proportion of women have symptoms before diagnosis.[1,2] The most common symptoms are vague and non-specific, resembling irritable bowel syndrome, and hence a diagnosis of ovarian cancer may be missed (Table 4.1). In general, further evaluation may be appropriate in a patient with severe or frequent symptoms of recent onset.[3]

Symptom indices have been developed in attempts to improve the sensitivity and specification of symptoms for the diagnosis of ovarian cancer. The most common of these is the Goff index,[1] which is considered positive if any of the following symptoms are present

TABLE 4.1

Common symptoms of ovarian cancer

- Abdominal bloating
- Increased abdominal size
- Changes in bowel function
- Constipation
- Early satiety
- Difficulty in eating
- Urinary complaints
- Pelvic pressure
- Pelvic or abdominal pain

more than 12 times a month but have developed within the previous 12 months:

- abdominal bloating or an increase in abdominal size
- difficulty in eating or feeling full
- pelvic or abdominal pain.

The Goff index has a sensitivity of approximately 67% for the diagnosis of ovarian cancer, and a specificity of approximately 90%.[1,2] However, the clinical usefulness of such indices depends on how the index is used (higher specificities are achieved when information about symptoms is obtained from clinical notes or questionnaires, rather than by telephone interview), and how index-positive patients are managed.[2]

The ongoing ROCkeTS (Refining Ovarian Cancer Test Accuracy Scores) study in the UK aims to validate risk prediction models that estimate the probability of having ovarian cancer for post- and premenopausal women with suspected ovarian cancer, and to define thresholds of predicted risk that inform decisions for patient management.[4]

Biomarkers. The most established biomarker for ovarian cancer is CA125, the levels of which mainly increase in the later stages of the disease. As a result, CA125 has only limited sensitivity (40–50%) for early-stage ovarian cancer.[4–6] A more recent tumor marker is the human epididymis secretory protein 4 (HE4), which is overexpressed in epithelial ovarian cancer.[7] This is used in combination with CA125 and menopausal status in the Risk of Ovarian Malignancy Algorithm (ROMA), which predicts the presence of ovarian cancer in patients with a pelvic mass, with a specificity and sensitivity of up to 95% and 76.4%, respectively;[8] specificity is higher in postmenopausal women. Over all ages, ROMA correctly classified 93.8% of patients with epithelial ovarian cancer as being at high risk.

Prospectively acquired evidence from the UK Collaborative Trial of Ovarian Cancer Screening (UKCTOCS) – which applied serial CA125 measurements interpreted via the Risk of Ovarian Cancer Algorithm (ROCA) – has shown that screening with this algorithm doubles the number of screen-detected epithelial ovarian cancers, compared with a fixed CA125 cut-off of 35 IU/mL. As a result, defined cut-offs need to be used with caution and always interpreted within the context of the whole clinical picture. A greater focus on interpreting trends in CA125 levels, along with the clinical picture and imaging findings, is likely to define the standard of care in the future.[9]

Imaging. The ability of current imaging techniques to accurately depict lesions in the peritoneum is limited, especially in fine nodular disease. This represents a significant challenge in diagnosing low-volume disease and accurately describing intra-abdominal tumor dissemination patterns. Nevertheless, CT has a well-established role in diagnosing bulky (> 1 cm) lymphadenopathy, distant intraparenchymatous metastatic lesions and additional lesions such as secondary cancers and thromboembolic events that have a significant effect on patient management.

Diffusion-weighted MRI may have a future role in the description of tumor dissemination patterns and assessment of operability, but prospective evidence data are needed.[10] There is also no evidence to support the routine use of positron emission tomography (PET)-CT, although this technique may be useful in highly specialized situations; for example, in the evaluation of thoracic or mediastinal lymph nodes before secondary or tertiary debulking.[11]

Staging

Complete surgical staging of ovarian cancer is essential to accurately define the stage of the disease and determine appropriate adjuvant treatment. This is a multistage process involving cytology, multiple peritoneal biopsies, omentectomy and, in cases of early disease, pelvic/para-aortic lymph node dissection (Figure 4.1). Up to 30% of patients with apparent early disease will be upstaged after comprehensive staging.[12]

The staging system of the International Federation of Gynecological Oncology (FIGO) is shown in Figure 4.2.[13] Having an accurate FIGO stage will influence the treatment strategies that are most appropriate for the individual patient.

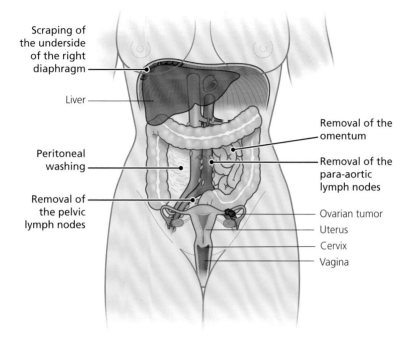

Scraping of the underside of the right diaphragm

Liver

Peritoneal washing

Removal of the pelvic lymph nodes

Removal of the omentum

Removal of the para-aortic lymph nodes

Ovarian tumor

Uterus

Cervix

Vagina

Figure 4.1 Complete surgical staging of ovarian cancer.

Grading

The grade of ovarian cancer reflects the degree of distortion from the normal tissue architecture and can correlate with aggressiveness and prognosis.

- Grade 1: well-differentiated tissue
- Grade 2: moderately differentiated tissue
- Grade 3: poorly differentiated tissue.

Serous tumors are often graded as high or low grade (see Chapter 2).

Stage I. Tumor confined to ovaries or fallopian tube(s)

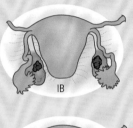

Uterus
Fallopian tube
Tumor
Ovary
IA

IA (T1a-N0-M0). Tumor limited to one ovary (capsule intact) or fallopian tube; no tumor on ovarian or fallopian tube surface; no malignant cells in the ascites or peritoneal washings

IB (T1b-N0-M0). Tumor limited to both ovaries (capsules intact) or fallopian tubes; no tumor on ovarian or fallopian tube surface; no malignant cells in the ascites or peritoneal washings

IB

IC1 (T1c-N0-M0). Tumor limited to one or both ovaries or fallopian tubes, with surgical spill

IC2 (T1c-N0-M0). Tumor limited to one or both ovaries or fallopian tubes, with capsule ruptured before surgery or tumor on ovarian or fallopian tube surface

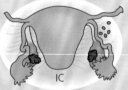

IC

IC3 (T1c-N0-M0). Tumor limited to one or both ovaries or fallopian tubes, with malignant cells in the ascites or peritoneal washings

Stage II. Tumor involves one or both ovaries or fallopian tubes with pelvic extension (below pelvic brim) or primary peritoneal cancer

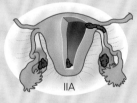

IIA

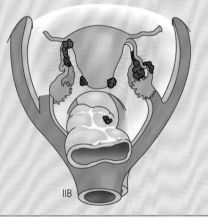

IIB

IIA (T2a-N0-M0). Extension and/or implants on uterus and/or fallopian tubes and/or ovaries

IIB (T2b-N0-M0). Extension to other pelvic intraperitoneal tissues

Stage III. Tumor involves one or both ovaries or fallopian tubes, or primary peritoneal cancer, with cytologically or histologically confirmed spread to the peritoneum outside the pelvis and/or metastasis to the retroperitoneal lymph nodes

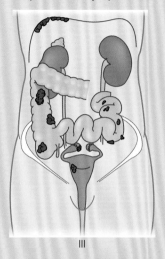

III

IIIA1 (T1/T2-N1-M0). Positive retroperitoneal lymph nodes only (cytologically or histologically proven)
  IIIA1(ii) Metastasis ≤ 10 mm
  IIIA1(iii) Metastasis > 10 mm
IIIA2 (T3a-N0/N1-M0). Microscopic extrapelvic (above the pelvic brim) peritoneal involvement with or without positive retroperitoneal lymph nodes
IIIB (T3b-N0/N1-M0). Macroscopic peritoneal metastasis beyond the pelvis ≤ 2 cm in greatest dimension, with or without metastasis to the retroperitoneal lymph nodes
IIIC (T3c-N0/N1-M0). Macroscopic peritoneal metastasis beyond the pelvis > 2 cm in greatest dimension, with or without metastasis to the retroperitoneal lymph nodes (includes extension of tumor to capsule of liver and spleen without parenchymal involvement of either organ)

Stage IV. Distant metastasis excluding peritoneal metastases

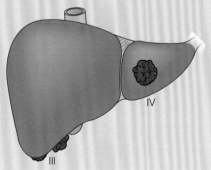

IV

III

IVA (Any T, any N, M1). Pleural effusion with positive cytology
IVB (Any T, any N, M1). Parenchymal metastases and metastases to extra-abdominal organs (including inguinal lymph nodes and lymph nodes outside of the abdominal cavity)

Figure 4.2 The FIGO staging system for ovarian, fallopian tube and peritoneal cancer. Tumor–nodes–metastases (TNM) stage is also shown. Adapted from www.ncbi.nlm.nih.gov/pmc/articles/PMC4397237/table/T1.

Key points – diagnosis, staging and grading

- The majority (> 80%) of women with epithelial ovarian cancer will become apparent and diagnosed at an advanced stage of the disease.
- There are no reliable imaging tools to accurately describe the stage of the disease or tumor dissemination patterns, especially in fine nodular peritoneal carcinomatosis and microscopically involved lymph nodes.
- Comprehensive surgical staging accurately defines the disease stage, resulting in more reliable prediction of prognosis and more appropriate management strategies and systemic treatment.

References

1 Lachance JA, Everett EN, Greer B et al. The effect of age on clinical/pathologic features, surgical morbidity, and outcome in patients with endometrial cancer. *Gynecol Oncol* 2006;101:470–5.

2 Lim AW, Mesher D, Gentry-Maharaj A et al. Predictive value of symptoms for ovarian cancer: comparison of symptoms reported by questionnaire, interview, and general practitioner notes. *J Natl Cancer Inst* 2012;104:114–24.

3 Goff BA, Mandel LS, Melancon CH, Muntz HG. Frequency of symptoms of ovarian cancer in women presenting to primary care clinics. *JAMA* 2004;291:2705–12.

4 Sundar S, Rick C, Dowling F et al. Refining Ovarian Cancer Test accuracy Scores (ROCkeTS): protocol for a prospective longitudinal test accuracy study to validate new risk scores in women with symptoms of suspected ovarian cancer. *BMJ Open* 2016;6:e010333.

5 Sagi-Dain L, Lavie O, Auslander R, Sagi S. CEA in evaluation of adnexal mass: retrospective cohort analysis and review of the literature. *Int J Biol Markers* 2015;30:e394–400.

6 Sagi-Dain L, Lavie O, Auslander R, Sagi S. CA 19–9 in evaluation of adnexal mass: retrospective cohort analysis and review of the literature. *Int J Biol Markers* 2015;30:e333–40.

7 Schummer M, Ng WV, Bumgarner RE et al. Comparative hybridization of an array of 21,500 ovarian cDNAs for the discovery of genes overexpressed in ovarian carcinomas. *Gene* 1999;238:375–85.

8 Moore RG, McMeekin DS, Brown AK et al. A novel multiple marker bioassay utilizing HE4 and CA125 for the prediction of ovarian cancer in patients with a pelvic mass. *Gynecol Oncol* 2009;112:40–6.

9 Menon U, Ryan A, Kalsi J et al. Risk algorithm using serial biomarker measurements doubles the number of screen-detected cancers compared with a single-threshold rule in the United Kingdom Collaborative Trial of Ovarian Cancer Screening. *J Clin Oncol* 2015;33:2062–71.

10 deSouza NM, Rockall A, Freeman S. Functional MR imaging in gynecologic cancer. *Magn Reson Imaging Clin N Am* 2016;24: 205–22.

11 Mapelli P, Incerti E, Fallanca F et al. Imaging biomarkers in ovarian cancer: the role of ^{18}F-FDG PET/CT. *Q J Nucl Med Mol Imaging* 2016;60:93–102.

12 Timmers PJ, Zwinderman AH, Coens C et al. Understanding the problem of inadequately staging early ovarian cancer. *Eur J Cancer* 2010;46:880–4.

13 Prat J, FIGO Committee on Gynecologic Oncology. Staging classification for cancer of the ovary, fallopian tube, and peritoneum. *Int J Gynaecol Obstet* 2014;124:1–5.

Further reading

Cannistra SA. Cancer of the ovary. *N Engl J Med* 2004;351:2519–29.

Trimbos JB. Surgical treatment of early-stage ovarian cancer. *Best Pract Res Clin Obstet Gynaecol* 2016;pii:S1521–6934(16)30094–3.

5 / Surgery

Surgery is the cornerstone of management for both early and advanced ovarian cancer, although the aims are different in each case.

- In patients with presumed early disease, the aim of surgery is to remove the primary tumor, along with adequate peritoneal and lymphogenic staging.
- In advanced disease, the aim is to achieve maximal cytoreduction and tumor reduction.

Surgery for primary ovarian cancer

Surgical management of primary ovarian cancer may involve non-fertility-sparing and fertility-sparing approaches (Figure 5.1).

Non-fertility-sparing surgery consists of cytological staging, removal of the ovaries, fallopian tubes and uterus, peritoneal biopsies and lymph node dissection (Table 5.1). In addition, appendicectomy should be considered in patients with mucinous histology, or if the appendix appears abnormal.[1,2]

TABLE 5.1

Stages of non-fertility-sparing surgery for ovarian cancer

- Cytology*
- Bilateral salpingo-oophorectomy
- Hysterectomy
- Multiple peritoneal biopsies from the paracolic spaces, and bilateral subdiaphragmatic spaces[†]
- Infragastric omentectomy
- Pelvic and bilateral para-aortic lymph node dissection to the level of the renal vessels

*Ideally taken before manipulation of the tumor.
[†]Even from normal appearing peritoneum.

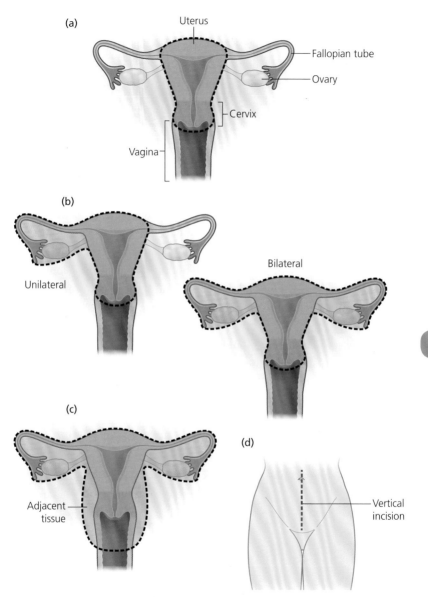

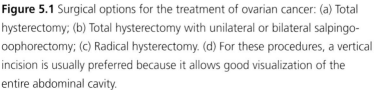

Figure 5.1 Surgical options for the treatment of ovarian cancer: (a) Total hysterectomy; (b) Total hysterectomy with unilateral or bilateral salpingo-oophorectomy; (c) Radical hysterectomy. (d) For these procedures, a vertical incision is usually preferred because it allows good visualization of the entire abdominal cavity.

Depending on the histological grade and tumor subtype, up to 30% of patients with apparently early epithelial ovarian cancer will be upstaged after comprehensive peritoneal and lymph node staging.[3–5] The only prospective randomized trial to have compared lymph node sampling alone with systematic lymph node dissection found that 13% of patients with lymph node involvement would be missed with lymph node sampling alone;[6] this clearly has important implications for tumor staging and choice of adjuvant treatment. However, in this study, systematic lymph node dissection was not associated with a significant survival benefit compared with sampling alone, partly because of a lack of statistical power but also because of common use of chemotherapy in the sampling arm, which seemed to potentially compensate for the less radical dissection. Increasing evidence shows that the prevalence of positive lymph nodes in stage IA mucinous cancer is extremely low, and that there is no value in performing surgery that can lead to unnecessary morbidity.[7,8]

Fertility-sparing surgery should be considered and discussed in younger patients and those with early-stage disease. Patients should be informed about the risks and benefits of such an approach, and the potentially higher risk of local relapse, which depends on their individual risk profile.

- Patients with stage IA ovarian cancer and favorable histology (low-grade mucinous, serous, endometrioid or mixed histology) have been shown to have a lower risk after fertility-preserving surgery than patients with a higher disease stage or tumor grade. In large retrospective analyses, women with grade 3 disease or stage IC3 with clear cell histology had a higher risk of recurrence (Figure 5.2), which was mainly related to the higher incidence of extra-ovarian spread in grade 3 tumors rather than to a higher relapse rate in the preserved ovary.[9] In retrospective studies, the risk of positive contralateral pelvic lymph nodes in women with unilateral disease despite negative ipsilateral nodes was as high as 11%.[5,6] For this reason, staging of pelvic lymph nodes should be bilateral.
- In advanced stages, maximal cytoreduction aimed at achieving complete tumor clearance has been shown to be associated with

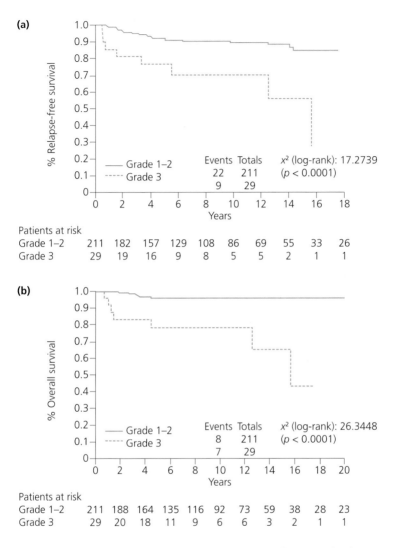

Figure 5.2 (a) Recurrence-free and (b) overall survival following fertility-sparing surgery for ovarian cancer according to tumor grade. Reproduced with permission from Fruscio R et al. 2013.[9]

significant increases in both overall and progression-free survival.[10–12] A meta-analysis of 53 studies and 6885 patients, from 1989 to 1998, showed that every 10% reduction in tumor was associated with a 6.3% prolongation of median overall survival.[13]

Resection techniques

In order to achieve total macroscopic tumor clearance in peritoneally disseminated disease, a maximal surgical effort is required, incorporating multivisceral resection techniques such as:

- extensive peritoneal stripping
- full thickness diaphragmatic resection
- removal of bulky pelvic/para-aortic lymph nodes
- splenectomy
- bowel resection.

Extra-abdominal cytoreductive procedures are increasingly being used to achieve complete tumor clearance outside the abdominal cavity. Techniques such as cardiophrenic/paracardiac lymph node dissection, pleurectomy, and supraclavicular and axillary lymph node dissection may be applied. Surgical expertise and training, with continuous audit of surgical outcome, morbidity and survival, have been proven to be important tools in making such extensive surgery safe for the patient without unnecessarily increasing morbidity.[14] For this reason, there is an increasing trend toward the use of such procedures only in specialized centers with adequate infrastructure, resources and training.

Pelvic and para-aortic lymph node dissection is part of the debulking procedure in patients with bulky lymph nodes. In a randomized Phase III trial, the removal of these nodes only, compared with systematic lymph node dissection, was associated with a reduction in 5-year progression-free survival rates (21.6% versus 31.2%, respectively), with no significant difference in overall survival.[15] Systematic pelvic and para-aortic lymphadenectomy offers no benefit in advanced disease in the absence of bulky lymph nodes.

Timing of surgery

Cytoreductive surgery for ovarian cancer is generally performed at the time of diagnosis, when it is referred to as primary cytoreduction. It is also performed during primary chemotherapy, when it is referred to as interval cytoreduction, and after disease recurrence, which is called secondary or tertiary cytoreduction.

The optimal timing of surgery in relation to first-line chemotherapy is still under debate. Two prospective randomized trials[12,16] have reported lower surgical morbidity and comparable survival when neoadjuvant therapy was given, compared with upfront surgery, but whether these findings can be generalized to patients with good performance status treated in specialized centers is unclear.

Ongoing trials (TRUST, AGO OVAR OP 7) are investigating the optimal timing of surgery, and will also address issues such as the optimal management of fragile patients.

Surgery for relapsed ovarian cancer

Despite the established value of cytoreduction in the primary tumor setting, the value of tumor debulking surgery for recurrent epithelial ovarian cancer is not well defined. These patients have a chronic condition and hence quality of life needs to be carefully balanced with the surgical risks.

Secondary cytoreduction. The DESKTOP I trial retrospectively evaluated the survival benefit of secondary debulking in patients with ovarian cancer, sensitive to platinum chemotherapy.[17] Complete tumor resection increased survival, compared with those with residual tumor (median 45.2 versus 19.7 months; hazard ratio [HR] 3.71, 95% confidence interval [CI] 2.27–6.05, $p < 0.0001$). Using these data, the Arbeitsgemeinschaft Gynaekologische Onkologie (AGO) determined that complete tumor resection was feasible in patients with recurrent disease provided they had:

• good performance status
• complete resection at primary surgery, or early FIGO stage (I/II)
• absence of gross ascites at relapse.

Patients that met all three of these criteria were given a positive AGO score.

An exploratory analysis of the DESKTOP results to evaluate the role of peritoneal carcinomatosis in recurrent epithelial ovarian cancer clearly showed that, even though peritoneal carcinomatosis was a negative predictor for complete resection in patients with recurrent disease, it appeared to have no independent negative impact on survival if total macroscopic clearance could be achieved.[17,18]

The prospective, multicenter DESKTOP II trial, subsequently validated the AGO score, confirming its usefulness and reliability for predicting the benefit of complete tumor resection in more than two-thirds of patients with platinum-sensitive relapsed epithelial ovarian cancer. Of 516 patients screened over 19 months, 261 (51%) were classified as AGO score-positive and 129 of them with first relapse underwent secondary tumor debulking. The rate of complete resection was 76%.[19] Interestingly, there was a poor correlation between imaging findings and intraoperative findings, both in terms of the number of lesions and localization of the tumor.

Perioperative morbidity and mortality appeared to be acceptable in the DESKTOP studies, with 0.8% mortality, 11% re-laparotomy (mainly due to bowel leakage or fistula in 7% of patients) and 2% deep vein thrombosis; 52% of patients required postoperative treatment in intensive care (median 2 days, range 1–20).

Similar findings have been reported in other patient series. A meta-analysis of data from 40 patients with recurrent epithelial ovarian cancer, spanning 24 years, showed that after controlling for all other disease-related factors, every 10% increase in the proportion of patients undergoing complete cytoreductive surgery was associated with a 3-month increase in median cohort survival time.[20]

Tertiary cytoreduction. The largest multicenter analysis of tertiary cytoreductive surgery evaluated 406 patients (median age 55 years; range 16–80) who underwent surgery between 1997 and 2011 in 12 centers across Europe, the USA and Asia.[21] Most of the patients had initial FIGO stage III/IV disease (69%), peritoneal carcinomatosis (51.7%) and absence of ascites (72.2%). The most frequent tumor dissemination site was the pelvis (73%). In total, 224 patients (54.1%) underwent complete tumor resection. This study confirmed that – even in the tertiary setting – complete macroscopic tumor clearance is a significant predictor of both overall and progression-free survival. Median overall survival for patients without residual tumor was

49 months (95% CI 42.5–56.4) compared with 12 months (95% CI 9.3–14.7) in patients with residual tumor ($p < 0.001$). By contrast, peritoneal carcinomatosis was not prognostic for survival after controlling for residual tumor status. Importantly, common clinicopathological characteristics such as tumor stage, age and histological subtype, which have been shown to be significant predictors of survival at initial presentation, did not appear to be of any prognostic significance at the tertiary stage. Multivariate analysis identified platinum resistance, residual tumor at secondary surgery and peritoneal carcinomatosis to be of predictive significance for complete tumor resection, while residual tumor at secondary and tertiary surgery, decreasing time to second relapse, ascites, upper abdominal tumor involvement and non-platinum third-line chemotherapy significantly affected overall survival.

A further clinically relevant finding was the significant impact of third-line postoperative systemic chemotherapy on overall survival, emphasizing the importance of a combination of systemic chemotherapy and surgical intervention, even in this heavily pretreated patient population. (This may reflect a selection bias, because those patients who were fit enough and able to tolerate chemotherapy following radical surgery may theoretically have had more favorable survival rates than patients who were too weak to tolerate any systemic treatment or in whom chemotherapy was contraindicated.)

Major operative morbidity and 30-day mortality rates were 25.9% and 3.2%, respectively; these are slightly higher than the equivalent data in the DESKTOP studies in the secondary treatment setting, but it should be noted that the study included both platinum-sensitive patients in whom cytoreduction was intended and symptomatic patients who underwent palliative surgery aimed at ameliorating their symptoms. The most common complication was infection/sepsis in 13% of patients; the re-laparotomy rate was 4.4%, but this was not associated with an increased risk of thromboembolic events (2.5%).

As in all surgical treatment for ovarian cancer, appropriate patient selection is crucial to minimize morbidity and maximize benefit from this radical approach.

Key points – surgery

- Surgery is one of the cornerstones of treatment for ovarian cancer.
- The key aims of surgery are tumor removal and accurate staging.
- Multivisceral surgery is needed to achieve complete tumor resection.
- Surgery for relapsed disease is associated with significant prolongation of progression-free survival in prospective studies; data for overall survival are not yet mature, but in retrospective series patients who are tumor free after surgery at relapse have significantly longer overall survival than those with residual tumor.
- Peritoneal carcinomatosis is associated with lower complete debulking rates at relapse, but not with inferior overall survival in tumor-free patients who undergo surgery.

References

1 Timmers PJ, Zwinderman K, Coens C et al. Lymph node sampling and taking of blind biopsies are important elements of the surgical staging of early ovarian cancer. *Int J Gynecol Cancer* 2010;20:1142–7.

2 Ledermann JA, Raja FA, Fotopoulou C et al. Newly diagnosed and relapsed epithelial ovarian carcinoma: ESMO clinical practice guidelines for diagnosis, treatment and follow-up. *Ann Oncol* 2013;24(Suppl 6):vi24–32.

3 Garcia-Soto AE, Boren T, Wingo SN et al. Is comprehensive surgical staging needed for thorough evaluation of early-stage ovarian carcinoma? *Am J Obstet Gynecol* 2012;206:242.e1–5.

4 Timmers PJ, Zwinderman AH, Coens C et al. Understanding the problem of inadequately staging early ovarian cancer. *Eur J Cancer* 2010;46:880–4.

5 Jayson GC, Kohn EC, Kitchener HC, Ledermann JA. Ovarian cancer. *Lancet* 2014;384:1376–88.

6 Maggioni A, Benedetti Panici P, Dell'Anna T et al. Randomised study of systematic lymphadenectomy in patients with epithelial ovarian cancer macroscopically confined to the pelvis. *Br J Cancer* 2006;95: 699–704.

7 Schmeler KM, Tao X, Frumovitz M et al. Prevalence of lymph node metastasis in primary mucinous carcinoma of the ovary. *Obstet Gynecol* 2010;116:269–73.

8 Kleppe M, Wang T, Van Gorp T et al. Lymph node metastasis in stages I and II ovarian cancer: a review. *Gynecol Oncol* 2011;123:610–14.

9 Fruscio R, Corso S, Ceppi L et al. Conservative management of early-stage epithelial ovarian cancer: results of a large retrospective series. *Ann Oncol* 2013;24:138–44.

10 du Bois A, Reuss A, Pujade-Lauraine E et al. Role of surgical outcome as prognostic factor in advanced epithelial ovarian cancer: a combined exploratory analysis of 3 prospectively randomized phase 3 multicenter trials: by the Arbeitsgemeinschaft Gynaekologische Onkologie Studiengruppe Ovarialkarzinom (AGO-OVAR) and the Groupe D'Investigateurs Nationaux Pour les Etudes des Cancers de L'Ovaire (GINECO). *Cancer* 2009;115: 1234–44.

11 van der Burg ME, van Lent M, Buyse M et al. The effect of debulking surgery after induction chemotherapy on the prognosis in advanced epithelial ovarian cancer. Gynecological Cancer Cooperative Group of the European Organization for Research and Treatment of Cancer. *N Engl J Med* 1995;332: 629–34.

12 Vergote I, Tropé CG, Amant F et al. Neoadjuvant chemotherapy or primary surgery in stage IIIC or IV ovarian cancer. *N Engl J Med* 2010;363:943–53.

13 Bristow RE, Tomacruz RS, Armstrong DK et al. Survival effect of maximal cytoreductive surgery for advanced ovarian carcinoma during the platinum era: a meta-analysis. *J Clin Oncol* 2002;20:1248–59.

14 Aletti GD, Gostout BS, Podratz KC, Cliby WA. Ovarian cancer surgical resectability: relative impact of disease, patient status, and surgeon. *Gynecol Oncol* 2006;100:33–7.

15 Panici PB, Maggioni A, Hacker N et al. Systematic aortic and pelvic lymphadenectomy versus resection of bulky nodes only in optimally debulked advanced ovarian cancer: a randomized clinical trial. *J Natl Cancer Inst* 2005;97:560–6.

16 Kehoe S, Hook J, Nankivell M et al. Primary chemotherapy versus primary surgery for newly diagnosed advanced ovarian cancer (CHORUS): an open-label, randomised, controlled, non-inferiority trial. *Lancet* 2015;386:249–57.

17 Harter P, du Bois A, Hahmann M et al. Surgery in recurrent ovarian cancer: the Arbeitsgemeinschaft Gynaekologische Onkologie (AGO) DESKTOP OVAR trial. *Ann Surg Oncol* 2006;13:1702–10.

18 Harter P, Hahmann M, Lueck HJ et al. Surgery for recurrent ovarian cancer: role of peritoneal carcinomatosis: exploratory analysis of the DESKTOP I trial about risk factors, surgical implications, and prognostic value of peritoneal carcinomatosis. *Ann Surg Oncol* 2009;16:1324–30.

19 Harter P, Sehouli J, Reuss A et al. Prospective validation study of a predictive score for operability of recurrent ovarian cancer: the Multicenter Intergroup Study DESKTOP II. A project of the AGO Kommission OVAR, AGO Study Group, NOGGO, AGO-Austria, and MITO. *Int J Gynecol Cancer* 2011;21:289–95.

20 Bristow RE, Puri I, Chi DS. Cytoreductive surgery for recurrent ovarian cancer: a meta-analysis. *Gynecol Oncol* 2009;112:265–74.

21 Fotopoulou C, Zang R, Gultekin M et al. Value of tertiary cytoreductive surgery in epithelial ovarian cancer: an international multicenter evaluation. *Ann Surg Oncol* 2013;20:1348–54.

Most patients with ovarian cancer present at advanced stages of disease, and thus require chemotherapy. Only those found to have stage I grade 1 disease after comprehensive staging are not considered for any adjuvant therapy. Patients with stage I grade 2 disease are sometimes excluded from adjuvant treatment, and the number of cycles prescribed is sometimes reduced in such cases. At least 6 cycles of chemotherapy are routinely recommended in patients with stage II disease and beyond (Figure 6.1).

Chemotherapy regimens

The adjuvant treatment of ovarian, fallopian tube and primary peritoneal cancers is complex in that multiple standards of care exist (Figure 6.2). Adjuvant approaches that are considered to be within current standards of care include:

- 'standard chemotherapy': platinum-based therapy (cisplatin or carboplatin) plus a taxane (paclitaxel or docetaxel) administered intravenously every 3 weeks
- 'dose-dense' chemotherapy: a platinum agent administered intravenously every 3 weeks with a weekly taxane
- weekly platinum plus taxane intravenous therapy
- neoadjuvant chemotherapy
- intraperitoneal (IP) chemotherapy: platinum and taxane administered intraperitoneally or intravenously
- standard chemotherapy with the addition of bevacizumab.

The choice of therapy depends on the physician, and is often tailored to the characteristics of the patient.

The combination of carboplatin and paclitaxel is the current standard of care for first-line chemotherapy in ovarian cancer. A number of key clinical trials have shown that a combination of paclitaxel and cisplatin is superior in efficacy to cisplatin plus cyclophosphamide,[1,2] and that carboplatin/paclitaxel is at least comparable in efficacy to cisplatin/paclitaxel but better tolerated (Table 6.1).[3,4]

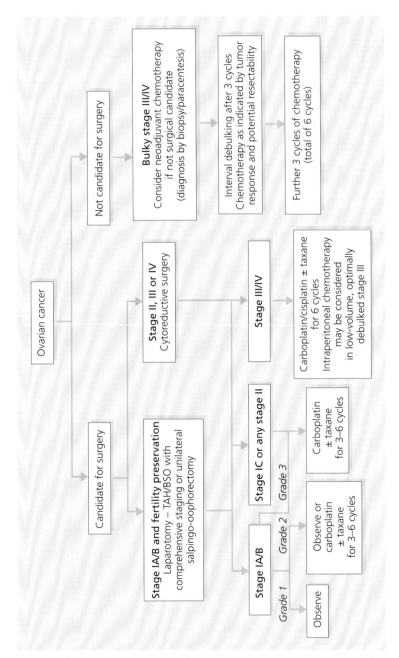

Figure 6.1 Management pathway for ovarian cancer according to stage of disease. TAH/BSO, total hysterectomy with bilaterial salpingo-oophorectomy.

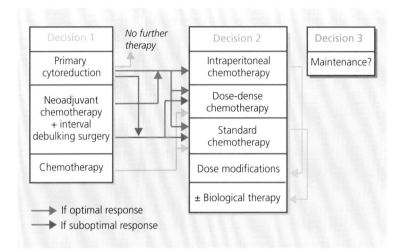

Figure 6.2 Key decisions with respect to treatment options for patients with advanced stage ovarian cancer.

TABLE 6.1

Key clinical trials that have defined the current standard of care for adjuvant chemotherapy in advanced ovarian cancer

Study	No. of patients	Key outcomes
Paclitaxel/cisplatin versus cyclophosphamide/cisplatin		
GOGIII[1]	384	PFS: 18 vs 13 months
		OS: 38 vs 24 months
EORTC-OV10[2]	680	PFS: 16 vs 12 months
		OS: 43 vs 44 months
Paclitaxel/carboplatin versus paclitaxel/cisplatin		
AGO[3]	798	PFS: 17 vs 19 months
		OS: 43 vs 44 months
GOG158[4]	792	PFS: 19 vs 21 months
		OS: 49 vs 57 months

AGO, Arbeitsgemeinschaft Gynäkologische Onkologie; EORTC, European Organisation for Research and Treatment of Cancer; GOG, Gynecologic Oncology Group; OS, overall survival; PFS, progression-free survival.

Adjuvant versus neoadjuvant therapy

As shown in Figure 6.2, the first treatment decision for patients with ovarian cancer is the timing of surgery. Many clinicians prefer to perform primary cytoreductive surgery initially, usually followed by 6 cycles of chemotherapy. The advantages of this approach include:

- establishing a definitive diagnosis
- removing the symptomatic tumor
- avoiding the theoretical concern of possibly inducing resistant clones by exposing large-volume tumors to chemotherapy.

However, other clinicians support the routine use of neoadjuvant chemotherapy, whereby chemotherapy is started after the diagnosis is established by biopsy, and surgery is performed after 3–4 cycles of chemotherapy have been administered. Most clinicians will opt for neoadjuvant therapy if the patient is judged to be a poor surgical risk, such as those of very advanced age, with significant comorbid conditions or who have a poor performance status.

Two landmark Phase III trials have shown that interval cytoreduction after initial chemotherapy is a viable option in patients with advanced stage ovarian cancer.[5,6] The first involved 670 women with stage IIIC/IV epithelial ovarian cancer, primary peritoneal cancer or fallopian tube cancer and an extrapelvic tumor 2 cm or more in diameter.[5] The experimental group received platinum-based neoadjuvant therapy, followed by interval debulking surgery and subsequent adjuvant chemotherapy; the control group received primary debulking surgery followed by at least 6 cycles of platinum-based chemotherapy. There were no significant differences between the study groups with regard to overall survival (OS) (hazard ratio [HR] 0.98; 90% CI 0.84–1.13, $p = 0.01$ for non-inferiority) or progression-free survival (PFS) (HR 1.01; 90% CI 0.89–1.15). However, there were significant differences between the study groups in the incidence of surgery-related serious (grade 3/4) adverse events, including hemorrhage (12 versus 23, respectively; relative risk [RR] 0.50; 95% CI 0.25–0.99), venous thromboembolism (0 versus 8; RR 0.06; 95% CI 0–0.98) and infection (5 versus 25; RR 0.19; 95% CI 0.07–0.50).

The second study (CHORUS) assigned 276 patients to primary surgery and 274 to primary chemotherapy.[6] Median OS was

22.6 months in the surgery group compared with 24.1 months in the chemotherapy group (HR for death 0·87 in favor of primary chemotherapy; 95% CI 0·72–1·05). Grade 3/4 postoperative adverse events and deaths within 28 days of surgery were more common in the surgery group than in the chemotherapy group (adverse events: 24% versus 14%, $p = 0.0007$; deaths: 6% versus < 1%, $p = 0·001$). The most common grade 3/4 postoperative adverse event in both groups was hemorrhage (3% versus 6% in the surgery and chemotherapy groups, respectively). Overall, 49% of women receiving primary surgery and 40% of those receiving primary chemotherapy had a grade 3/4 chemotherapy-related adverse event, mostly uncomplicated neutropenia (20% and 16%, respectively). The authors concluded that neoadjuvant chemotherapy was not inferior to primary debulking surgery, and that administration of chemotherapy before surgery is an acceptable standard of care for women with advanced ovarian cancer.

As a result of these studies, the Society of Gynecologic Oncology (SGO) and the American Society of Clinical Oncology (ASCO) issued a joint guidance statement on the use of neoadjuvant chemotherapy in patients with advanced ovarian cancer.[7] Key recommendations from these guidelines are summarized in Table 6.2.

TABLE 6.2

Key recommendations from the SGO/ASCO guidelines on the use of neoadjuvant chemotherapy in women with advanced ovarian cancer[7]

All women with advanced ovarian cancer should be evaluated by a gynecologic oncologist to determine whether primary or interval cytoreduction is most appropriate.

Women who have a high perioperative risk profile or a low likelihood of achieving cytoreduction to < 1 cm (ideally to no visible disease) should receive neoadjuvant chemotherapy.

For women with a high likelihood of achieving cytoreduction to < 1 cm (ideally to no visible disease) with acceptable morbidity, primary cytoreduction is recommended over neoadjuvant chemotherapy.

ASCO, American Society of Clinical Oncology; SGO, Society of Gynecologic Oncology.

According to these guidelines, a key component in the choice of adjuvant or neoadjuvant therapy (in addition to patient comorbidities) is the ability to cytoreduce, based upon tumor distribution. The goal is to cytoreduce to no gross residual tumor, as this R–0 status yields the highest survival rates.

Choice of adjuvant therapy regimen

Dose-dense regimens. If adjuvant therapy is chosen, the second key decision (see Figure 6.2) is the selection of dose schedule. The standard regimen usually comprises carboplatin, at a dose intended to achieve an area under the curve (AUC) of 5–7.5 mg/mL/minute, and paclitaxel, 175 mg/m^2. However, some investigators have explored a 'dose-dense' approach, whereby higher doses are administered over a shorter period of time. Adapting favorable efficacy data from the breast cancer literature, most such approaches have involved changes in the paclitaxel dose schedule, with administration on a weekly basis rather than every 3 weeks, at a dose of 80 mg/m^2. A large Phase III randomized trial showed superiority for this dose-dense approach using the weekly paclitaxel schedule.[8,9]

The MITO 7 study explored the possibility of fractionating the doses of both the platinum and taxane components.[10] There was no statistically significant advantage in terms of OS or PFS compared with standard therapy, but the paclitaxel dose (60 mg/m^2) was lower than that normally used in dose-dense regimens. Neuropathy and hair loss were reduced in the dose-dense or weekly approach. More recently, the GOG262 study,[11] which explored the dose-dense approach versus 3-weekly paclitaxel with the option of bevacizumab administration, showed no advantage in terms of PFS with dose-dense therapy; however, in a post hoc analysis of the group who opted not to receive bevacizumab (approximately 15% of the population), there was a statistically significant difference in PFS favoring dose-dense chemotherapy.

Concomitant anti-angiogenesis treatment. Two large Phase III trials that explored the concept of adding bevacizumab to front-line treatment for ovarian cancer met their primary endpoint of improving

PFS, but neither showed an improvement in OS.[12,13] The use of bevacizumab in this setting varies between countries, depending on the licensed indications for the drug in each country.

Intraperitoneal chemotherapy. The use of IP chemotherapy has been advocated for small-volume residual disease, given that an extremely high peritoneal to serum drug concentration ratio can potentially be achieved by this approach. Several randomized studies have shown that IP therapy can produce improvements of 20–30% in PFS, OS, or both (Table 6.3).[14–17] However, to date the GOG252 trial has not shown an advantage for IP therapy in terms of the primary endpoint, PFS;[17] it has been suggested that the lower doses of drug used in this study, and the use of bevacizumab in all three arms of the trial, may have confounded the efficacy results.

Increased toxicity is an important concern in patients receiving IP chemotherapy. For example, in the GOG172 trial, which compared intravenous and IP paclitaxel and cisplatin, grade 3/4 fatigue, pain or hematologic, gastrointestinal, metabolic or neurological toxicities were significantly more common with IP than with intravenous therapy (Table 6.4).[16]

TABLE 6.3

Efficacy of intraperitoneal chemotherapy in randomized studies in patients with advanced stage ovarian cancer

	Median PFS (months)		% increase	Median OS (months)		% increase
	IV	IP		IV	IP	
SWOG/ GOG104[14]	NR	NR		41	49	20%
GOG114[15]	22	28	27%	52	63	21%
GOG172[16]	18	24	26%	50	67	29%
GOG252[17]	27	29	28 NS	Pending	Pending	

GOG, Gynecologic Oncology Group; IP, intraperitoneal; IV, intravenous; NR, not reported. NS, not significant; OS, overall survival; PFS, progression-free survival; SWOG, originally known as the Southwest Oncology Group.

TABLE 6.4

Incidence of grade 3/4 adverse events in the GOG172 trial of intraperitoneal (IP) versus intravenous (IV) cisplatin and paclitaxel chemotherapy[16]

Adverse event	IV therapy (n = 210)	IP therapy (n = 201)	Significance
Leukopenia*	134 (64%)	152 (76%)	$p < 0.001$
Platelet count < 25 000/mm³	8 (4%)	24 (12%)	$p = 0.002$
Other hematologic	190 (90%)	188 (94%)	$p = 0.87$
Gastrointestinal	51 (24%)	92 (46%)	$p < 0.001$
Renal/genitourinary	5 (2%)	14 (7%)	$p = 0.03$
Pulmonary	5 (2%)	7 (3%)	$p = 0.50$
Cardiovascular	10 (5%)	19 (9%)	$p = 0.06$
Neurological	18 (9%)	39 (19%)	$p = 0.001$
Cutaneous changes	2 (1%)	2 (1%)	$p = 0.96$
Lymphatic system	0 (0%)	3 (1%)	$p = 0.07$
Fever	8 (4%)	19 (9%)	$p = 0.02$
Infection	2 (6%)	33 (16%)	$p = 0.001$
Fatigue	9 (4%)	36 (18%)	$p < 0.001$
Metabolic	15 (7%)	55 (27%)	$p < 0.001$
Pain	3 (1%)	23 (11%)	$p < 0.001$
Hepatic	1 (< 1%)	6 (3%)	$p = 0.05$
Other	1 (< 1%)	6 (3%)	$p = 0.05$

*White cell count < 1000/mm³.

Among the current standards of care, the choice of therapy is generally based on a number of considerations, including:

- patient characteristics (age, performance status, comorbidities, etc.)
- physician preference
- regulatory approval
- reimbursement considerations
- regional variation.

The key data and other considerations shaping the choice between regimens are depicted in Figure 6.3. Future trials exploring long-term efficacy and toxicity in addition to patient-reported outcomes, such as quality of life, are likely to further clarify the value of each regimen. In addition, future trials will examine novel combinations of targeted agents with traditional chemotherapy.

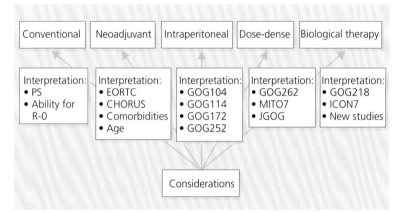

Figure 6.3 Key trials and other factors influencing the choice of adjuvant chemotherapy in advanced stage ovarian cancer. EORTC, European Organisation for Research and Treatment of Cancer; GOG, Gynecologic Oncology Group; ICON, International Collaborative Ovarian Neoplasm (study); JGOG, Japanese Gynecologic Oncology Group; MITO, Multicentre Italian Trials in Ovarian Cancer (study group); PS, performance status; R-0, no gross residual disease.

Key points – chemotherapy

- Most patients with ovarian cancer present at advanced stages of disease, and thus require chemotherapy.
- The combination of carboplatin and paclitaxel is the standard of care for the front-line treatment of ovarian cancer.
- Options for adjuvant therapy include standard chemotherapy, dose-dense chemotherapy and intraperitoneal treatment.
- A key component in the choice of adjuvant or neoadjuvant therapy is the ability to cytoreduce, ideally to 'no gross residual tumor'.
- Women who have a high perioperative risk profile or a low likelihood of achieving cytoreduction to less than 1 cm (ideally to no visible disease) should receive neoadjuvant chemotherapy.
- Among the current standards of care, the choice of therapy is generally based on a number of considerations, including patient characteristics, physician preference and regulatory status.

References

1 McGuire WP, Hoskins WJ, Brady MF et al. Cyclophosphamide and cisplatin compared with paclitaxel and cisplatin in patients with stage III and stage IV ovarian cancer. *N Engl J Med* 1996;334:1–6.

2 Piccart MJ, Bertelsen K, James K et al. Randomized intergroup trial of cisplatin-paclitaxel versus cisplatin-cyclophosphamide in women with advanced epithelial ovarian cancer: three-year results. *J Natl Cancer Inst* 2000;92:699–708.

3 du Bois A, Lück HJ, Meier W et al.; Arbeitsgemeinschaft Gynäkologische Onkologie Ovarian Cancer Study Group. A randomized clinical trial of cisplatin/paclitaxel versus carboplatin/paclitaxel as first-line treatment of ovarian cancer. *J Natl Cancer Inst* 2003;95:1320–9.

4 Ozols RF, Bundy BN, Greer BE et al.; Gynecologic Oncology Group. Phase III trial of carboplatin and paclitaxel compared with cisplatin and paclitaxel in patients with optimally resected stage III ovarian cancer: a Gynecologic Oncology Group study. *J Clin Oncol* 2003;21:3194–200.

5 Vergote I, Tropé CG, Amant F et al.; European Organization for Research and Treatment of Cancer-Gynaecological Cancer Group, NCIC Clinical Trials Group. Neoadjuvant chemotherapy or primary surgery in stage IIIC or IV ovarian cancer. *N Engl J Med* 2010;363:943–53.

6 Kehoe S, Hook J, Nankivell M et al. Primary chemotherapy versus primary surgery for newly diagnosed advanced ovarian cancer (CHORUS): an open-label, randomised, controlled, non-inferiority trial. *Lancet* 2015;386:249–57.

7 Wright AA, Bohlke K, Armstrong DK et al. Neoadjuvant chemotherapy for newly diagnosed, advanced ovarian cancer: Society of Gynecologic Oncology and American Society of Clinical Oncology Clinical Practice Guideline. *J Clin Oncol* 2016;34:3460–73.

8 Fujiwara K, Aotani E, Hamano T et al. A randomized Phase II/III trial of 3 weekly intraperitoneal versus intravenous carboplatin in combination with intravenous weekly dose-dense paclitaxel for newly diagnosed ovarian, fallopian tube and primary peritoneal cancer. *Jpn J Clin Oncol* 2011;41:278–82.

9 Katsumata N, Yasuda M, Isonishi S et al.; Japanese Gynecologic Oncology Group. Long-term results of dose-dense paclitaxel and carboplatin versus conventional paclitaxel and carboplatin for treatment of advanced epithelial ovarian, fallopian tube, or primary peritoneal cancer (JGOG 3016): a randomised, controlled, open-label trial. *Lancet Oncol* 2013;14:1020–6.

10 Pignata S, Scambia G, Katsaros D et al.; Multicentre Italian Trials in Ovarian cancer (MITO–7), Groupe D'Investigateurs Nationaux pour L'Etude des Cancers Ovariens et du sein (GINECO), Mario Negri Gynecologic Oncology (MaNGO), European Network of Gynaecological Oncological Trial Groups (ENGOT-OV–10), Gynecologic Cancer InterGroup (GCIG) investigators. Carboplatin plus paclitaxel once a week versus every 3 weeks in patients with advanced ovarian cancer (MITO–7): a randomised, multicentre, open-label, phase 3 trial. *Lancet Oncol* 2014;15:396–405.

11 Chan JK, Brady MF, Penson RT et al. Weekly vs. every-3-week paclitaxel and carboplatin for ovarian cancer. *N Engl J Med* 2016;374:738–48.

12 Burger RA, Brady MF, Bookman MA et al.; Gynecologic Oncology Group. Incorporation of bevacizumab in the primary treatment of ovarian cancer. *N Engl J Med* 2011;365:2473–83.

13 Perren TJ, Swart AM, Pfisterer J et al.; ICON7 investigators. A phase 3 trial of bevacizumab in ovarian cancer. *N Engl J Med* 2011;365:2484–96.

14 Alberts DS, Liu PY, Hannigan EV et al. Intraperitoneal cisplatin plus intravenous cyclophosphamide versus intravenous cisplatin plus intravenous cyclophosphamide for stage III ovarian cancer. *N Engl J Med* 1996;335:1950–5.

15 Markman M, Bundy BN, Alberts DS et al. Phase III trial of standard-dose intravenous cisplatin plus paclitaxel versus moderately high-dose carboplatin followed by intravenous paclitaxel and intraperitoneal cisplatin in small-volume stage III ovarian carcinoma: an intergroup study of the Gynecologic Oncology Group, Southwestern Oncology Group, and Eastern Cooperative Oncology Group. *J Clin Oncol* 2001;19: 1001–7.

16 Armstrong DK, Bundy B, Wenzel L et al.; Gynecologic Oncology Group. Intraperitoneal cisplatin and paclitaxel in ovarian cancer. *N Engl J Med* 2006;354:34–43.

17 Walker JL, Brady MF, DiSilvestro PA et al. A Phase III clinical trial of bevacizumab with IV versus IP chemotherapy in ovarian, fallopian tube and primary peritoneal carcinoma NCI-supplied agent(s): bevacizumab (NSC#704865, IND#7921) NCT01167712 a GOG/NRG trial (GOG 252). Presented at the 2016 meeting of the American Society of Clinical Oncology, 03–07 June 2016, Chicago, Illinois, USA.

Further reading

Herzog TJ, Cohn DE. Dose dense chemotherapy for front-line ovarian cancer treatment: the price is right? *Gynecol Oncol* 2017;145:1–2.

Despite initial treatment, ovarian cancer will recur in nearly two-thirds of women who originally presented with advanced disease. In this situation, the aims of treatment change from achieving cure to:

- extending survival
- preserving quality of life by mitigating treatment-related adverse effects and ameliorating symptoms of the recurrent disease.

Surveillance

Recurrent ovarian cancer may present in a number of ways, and may be asymptomatic or symptomatic. With asymptomatic (chemical) recurrence, disease may be minimal and the value of treatment in this situation has been challenged. The use of routine CA125 monitoring after front-line therapy varies globally, and is still common in the USA despite data questioning the value of such monitoring.[1]

Imaging studies may be ordered if CA125 is not used to monitor for recurrence, but this approach is costly and exposes the patient to significant radiation over time. Furthermore, the sensitivity and specificity of imaging is suboptimal in ovarian cancer, because patients often exhibit numerous postsurgical changes; moreover, recurrences can occur with small-volume disease. Many clinicians reserve imaging for patients who present with symptoms or physical examination findings that are suggestive of recurrence.

Some patients with recurrent ovarian cancer may present with abdominal symptoms such as bloating, early satiety, pain or a change in urinary or bowel habits, or with more systemic symptoms such as fatigue. Elevated CA125, or other tumor markers such as human epididymis secretory protein 4 (HE4), may be confirmatory, along with imaging.

Treatment

The choice of treatment in patients with recurrent ovarian cancer will depend on a number of patient-, drug- and tumor-related factors (Figure 7.1). Traditionally, the choice of treatment has been determined

63

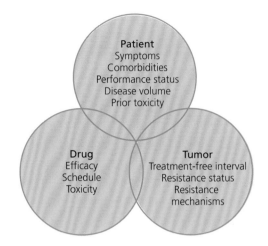

Figure 7.1 Patient-, drug- and tumor-related factors to take into consideration before treating recurrent ovarian cancer.

by the time that has elapsed since the last platinum-based chemotherapy: in practice, however, the treatment-free interval, irrespective of last platinum dose, may be even more valuable. In the near future, these somewhat restrictive determinants of treatment will be supplemented with more predictive factors such as *BRCA* status or tumor histology, and by gene- or pathway-based assessments that facilitate individualized therapy.[2] Nevertheless, the traditional definitions of platinum resistance or sensitivity remain relevant in guiding treatment (Figure 7.2).

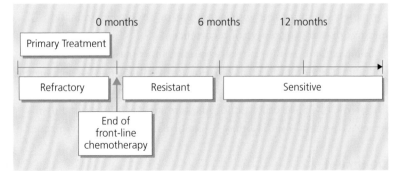

Figure 7.2 Timeline of treatment for recurrent ovarian cancer. Platinum sensitivity is classified as refractory, resistant or sensitive, according to the time that has elapsed since finishing front-line platinum chemotherapy.

Platinum-sensitive patients are generally treated with platinum-containing regimens. Recent trials with poly (ADP-ribose) polymerase (PARP) inhibitors have introduced the concept of switch maintenance, whereby a PARP inhibitor is used for those who are responding to subsequent platinum-based therapies (see pages 74–7).

Patients in whom recurrence occurs more than 6 months after primary platinum treatment are often subdivided into two groups:

- highly platinum-sensitive patients, in whom recurrence occurs more than 12 months after primary platinum treatment
- intermediately sensitive patients, in whom recurrence occurs 6–12 months after primary treatment.

Platinum-resistant patients, in whom recurrence occurs within 6 months of primary platinum treatment, are generally treated with non-platinum options; these usually include single agent chemotherapies with or without bevacizumab. Some clinicians define patients who actually progress on front-line treatment as platinum-refractory. They are often treated similarly to platinum-resistant patients, although some clinicians recommend continuing the platinum backbone while substituting the taxane with an alternative chemotherapeutic.

The prognosis and probability of response to subsequent treatment correlate directly with the time from the previous platinum or other treatment (Figure 7.3).

It should be emphasized that any patient who can potentially participate in a clinical trial should be offered this option as the preferred treatment.

Chemotherapy for platinum-sensitive disease. The initial treatment decision for a patient with platinum-sensitive disease is whether or not to perform surgery (see page 54). Chemotherapy options for platinum-sensitive disease have continued to expand. Such patients are actively recruited for clinical trials, because this population is widely believed to show a good balance between performance status, time to recurrence and potential for response to therapy. Many platinum-sensitive patients will respond to numerous regimens; as described above, some clinicians treat patients with recurrence at 6–12 months differently to those with

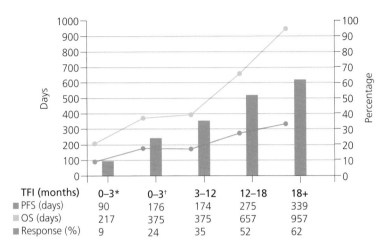

TFI (months)	0–3*	0–3†	3–12	12–18	18+
■ PFS (days)	90	176	174	275	339
▨ OS (days)	217	375	375	657	957
■ Response (%)	9	24	35	52	62

Figure 7.3 Relationship between treatment-free interval (TFI) and survival in recurrent ovarian cancer. *Progressive disease (refractory). †Non-progressive disease (partial response). OS, overall survival; PFS, progression-free survival.[3,4]

recurrence more than 12 months after previous platinum treatment. This is especially true when the recurrence is close to the 6-month cut-off, because many such patients have a response and prognosis similar to those who are platinum-resistant.

Typically, platinum is combined with either a taxane, pegylated liposomal doxorubicin (PLD) or gemcitabine. The choice of combination depends on several factors. For example, cumulative toxicities such as neuropathy can preclude retreatment with taxanes, and an alternative with a different mechanism of action, such as PLD or gemcitabine, may be preferred if the time from the previous platinum and taxane has been short. Key Phase III clinical trials with chemotherapy in patients with platinum-sensitive recurrent disease are summarized in Table 7.1.

Biological therapy for platinum-sensitive disease. Bevacizumab represents another option for platinum-sensitive patients. The OCEANS trial showed a significant improvement in progression-free survival (PFS) among those treated with bevacizumab, compared with placebo, when combined with carboplatin/gemcitabine.[8] Other studies have shown that bevacizumab can be combined with carboplatin/PLD

TABLE 7.1

Key Phase III trials in patients with platinum-sensitive recurrent ovarian cancer

Trial	Intervention	n	Progression-free survival (months)	Overall survival (months)
ICON4[5]	Platinum ± paclitaxel	802	9.0 vs 12.0 (HR 0.76, $p < 0.001$)	24 vs 29 (HR 0.82, $p = 0.02$)
AGO-OVAR–2.5[6]	Carboplatin ± gemcitabine	366	5.8 vs 8.6 (HR 0.72, $p = 0.003$)	17.3 vs 18.0 (HR 0.96, NS)
CALYPSO[7]	Carboplatin + paclitaxel Carboplatin + PLD	976	9.4 vs 11.3 months (HR 0.82, $p = 0.005$)	31.5 months (HR 0.99, NS)
OCEANS[8]	Carboplatin/ gemcitabine ± bevacizumab	484	8.4 vs 12.4 (HR 0.48, $p < 0.0001$)	35.2 vs 33.3 (HR 1.03, NS; immature data)
GOG213[9]	Carboplatin/ paclitaxel ± bevacizumab	673	10.4 vs 13.8 (HR 0.61, $p < 0.0001$)	37.3 vs 42.6 (HR 0.84, $p = 0.056$)

HR, hazard ratio; NS, not significant; PLD, pegylated liposomal doxorubicin.

or carboplatin/paclitaxel. Recently, the GOG213 study reported a significant improvement in PFS in patients treated with carboplatin/paclitaxel plus bevacizumab, compared with chemotherapy alone (median PFS 13.8 months versus 10.4 months, respectively, HR: 0.61, $p < 0.0001$); there was also a trend toward a significant improvement in overall survival (OS) (median 5.3 months increase, $p = 0.056$), which became statistically significant upon sensitivity analysis ($p = 0.0447$).[9] Bevacizumab increased the rate of hypertension requiring medical intervention from 1% to 12%, but the rate of gastrointestinal wall disruption did not change significantly (control 1% versus bevacizumab 2%).

As discussed in Chapter 8, PARP inhibitors confer an excellent response in platinum-sensitive patients, and their role appears to be expanding beyond patients with biomarkers such as *BRCA* mutations. The challenge for clinicians will be to decide upon the best use of these agents as either treatment or maintenance options in platinum-sensitive patients.

Chemotherapy for platinum-resistant disease. Patients with disease that recurs within 6 months of primary platinum treatment are generally treated with single agents, with or without bevacizumab. The most commonly used agents for retreatment include (usually weekly) paclitaxel, docetaxel, PLD, gemcitabine, topotecan and pemetrexed. Key clinical trials with these agents are summarized in Table 7.2. Unfortunately, the survival data and the objective response rates (less than 15%) are not impressive for any of the available single agents in the platinum-resistant setting; novel compounds and approaches are needed.

An important decision for clinicians is how best to use bevacizumab for the treatment of ovarian cancer. In some regions, bevacizumab is used in the front-line setting, while in others it is restricted to platinum-sensitive patients. Both the AURELIA trial in platinum-resistant patients,[13] and the OCEANS trial in platinum-sensitive patients,[8] yielded identical hazard ratios of 0.48 for PFS. Importantly, factors such as the presence of ascites or effusions, potential bowel toxicity with later lines, response or toxicity in earlier lines and affordability need to be considered in optimizing the use of bevacizumab.

Surgery. Although the value of tumor debulking surgery is well established for the treatment of primary tumors, the value of cytoreduction for recurrent epithelial ovarian cancer is not well defined. Appropriate patient selection is crucial (see Chapter 5).

TABLE 7.2

Key Phase III trials in patients with platinum-resistant recurrent ovarian cancer

Study	Intervention	n	PFS (mo)	OS (mo)	Comments
NCT-00113607 (subgroup analysis)[10,11]	PLD ± trabectedin	228	3.7 vs 4.0 (HR 0.95, NS)	14.2 vs 12.4 (HR 0.92, NS)	Response rate 16% vs 23%
TRINOVA–1 (subgroup analysis)[12]	Weekly paclitaxel ± trebananib	480	5.6 vs 3.8 (HR 0.66, $p < 0.001$)	18.3 vs 19.3 (HR 0.95, NS)	Effect on OS in patients with ascites
AURELIA[13]	Chemotherapy (weekly paclitaxel, gemcitabine, topotecan) ± bevacizumab	361	3.4 vs 6.7 (HR 0.48, $p < 0.001$)	16.6 vs 13.3 (HR 0.85, NS)	Response rate by RECIST: 12% vs 27%
AGO-OVAR 2.20/ ENGOT-ov14/ PENELOPE[14]	Chemotherapy (weekly paclitaxel, gemcitabine, topotecan) ± pertuzumab	156	4.3 vs 2.6 (HR 0.74, NS)	10.3 vs 7.9 (HR 0.84, NS)	All patients had low HER3 expression

HER3, human epidermal growth factor receptor 3; HR, hazard ratio; mo, months; NS, not significant; OS, overall survival; PFS, progression-free survival; RECIST, Response Evaluation Criteria In Solid Tumors.

Key points – recurrent ovarian cancer

- Ovarian cancer will recur in approximately two-thirds of patients with advanced ovarian cancer after primary treatment.
- The choice of treatment in patients with recurrent ovarian cancer will depend on a number of patient-, drug- and tumor-related factors.
- Platinum-sensitive patients are generally treated with platinum-containing regimens. Platinum-resistant patients are generally treated with non-platinum single agent chemotherapies with or without bevacizumab.
- Survival data and response rates are suboptimal with all single-agent therapies used in platinum-resistant recurrent disease: new therapies are needed in this setting.

References

1 Rustin GJ, van der Burg ME, Griffin CL et al. Early versus delayed treatment of relapsed ovarian cancer (MRC OV05/EORTC 55955): a randomised trial. *Lancet* 2010;376:1155–63.

2 Alvarez RD, Matulonis UA, Herzog TJ et al. Moving beyond the platinum sensitive/resistant paradigm for patients with recurrent ovarian cancer. *Gynecol Oncol* 2016;141:405–9.

3 Pujade-Lauraine E. Predicting the effectiveness of chemotherapy (Cx) in patients with recurrent ovarian cancer (ROC): a GINECO study. Presented at the 38th Annual Meeting of the American Society of Clinical Oncology (ASCO), 18–21 May 2002, Orlando, Florida, USA. Abstract 829.

4. Monk B, Coleman R. Changing the paradigm in the treatment of platinum-sensitive recurrent ovarian cancer: from platinum doublets to nonplatinum doublets and adding antiangiogenesis compounds. *Int J Gynecol Cancer* 2009;19: S63–7.

5 Parmar MK, Ledermann JA, Colombo N et al. Paclitaxel plus platinum-based chemotherapy versus conventional platinum-based chemotherapy in women with relapsed ovarian cancer: the ICON4/AGO-OVAR–2.2 trial. *Lancet* 2003;361:2099–106.

6 Pfisterer J, Plante M, Vergote I et al. Gemcitabine plus carboplatin compared with carboplatin in patients with platinum-sensitive recurrent ovarian cancer: an intergroup trial of the AGO-OVAR, the NCIC CTG, and the EORTC GCG. *J Clin Oncol* 2006;24: 4699–707.

7 Pujade-Lauraine E, Wagner U, Aavall-Lundqvist E et al. Pegylated liposomal doxorubicin and carboplatin compared with paclitaxel and carboplatin for patients with platinum-sensitive ovarian cancer in late relapse. *J Clin Oncol* 2010;28:3323–9.

8 Aghajanian C, Blank SV, Goff BA et al. OCEANS: a randomized, double-blind, placebo-controlled phase III trial of chemotherapy with or without bevacizumab in patients with platinum-sensitive recurrent epithelial ovarian, primary peritoneal, or fallopian tube cancer. *J Clin Oncol* 2012;30:2039–45.

9 Basen-Engquist K, Huang HQ, Herzog TJ et al. Randomized phase III trial of carboplatin/paclitaxel alone (CP) or in combination with bevacizumab followed by bevacizumab (CPB) and secondary cytoreduction surgery in platinum-sensitive recurrent ovarian cancer: GOG0213, an NRG Oncology/GOG study – analysis of patient reported outcomes (PRO) on chemotherapy randomization. *J Clin Oncol* 2015(suppl; abstr. 5525).

10 Monk BJ, Herzog TJ, Kaye SB et al. Trabectedin plus pegylated liposomal doxorubicin in recurrent ovarian cancer. *J Clin Oncol* 2010;28:3107–14.

11 Monk BJ, Herzog TJ, Kaye SB et al. Trabectedin plus pegylated liposomal doxorubicin (PLD) versus PLD in recurrent ovarian cancer: overall survival analysis. *Eur J Cancer* 2012;48:2361–8.

12 Monk BJ, Poveda A, Vergote I et al. Anti-angiopoietin therapy with trebananib for recurrent ovarian cancer (TRINOVA–1): a randomised, multicentre, double-blind, placebo-controlled phase 3 trial. *Lancet Oncol* 2014;15: 799–808.

13 Pujade-Lauraine E, Hilpert F, Weber B et al. Bevacizumab combined with chemotherapy for platinum-resistant recurrent ovarian cancer: the AURELIA open-label randomized phase III trial. *J Clin Oncol* 2014;32:1302–8.

14 Kurzeder C, Bover I, Marmé F et al. Double-blind, placebo-controlled, randomized phase III trial evaluating pertuzumab combined with chemotherapy for low tumor human epidermal growth factor receptor 3 mRNA-expressing platinum-resistant ovarian cancer (PENELOPE). *J Clin Oncol* 2016;34:2516–25.

8 Targeted therapies

There remain a number of unmet medical needs in the treatment of ovarian cancer, including improving cure rates and overcoming acquired resistance to platinum. Despite the availability of a number of new chemotherapies in both front-line and recurrent disease, cure rates have improved only modestly over the past few decades. Clearly, novel approaches are needed that exploit critical oncogenic pathways controlling tumor proliferation, angiogenesis, metastasis and apoptosis.

Precision medicine has become a key strategy in ovarian cancer as a result of advances in a number of areas, including pharmacogenomics, bioinformatics and molecular biology (Figure 8.1). It is hoped that precision medicine will allow the identification of patients who could maximally benefit from a particular drug or combination of drugs, and that this more precise targeted strategy will result in improved efficacy while minimizing toxicity.

Ultimately, it is hoped that targeted therapies will offer improved outcomes.

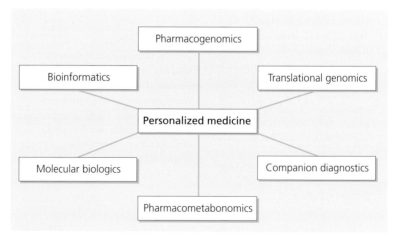

Figure 8.1. The multifaceted development of personalized (targeted) therapy in ovarian cancer.

Approaches to targeted therapy

The first attempts at developing targeted therapies in ovarian cancer have revolved around the recognition that epithelial ovarian cancers have different prognoses and distinct molecular changes associated with different histological subtypes.[1] Among the tumors with a better prognostic histology, high-grade serous carcinomas (HGSC) commonly present with *p53* mutations and overall genomic instability, while endometrioid tumors often exhibit *PTEN* and *PI3K* mutations. By contrast, mucinous and clear cell tumors confer a significantly worse prognosis, and are more usually associated with *KRAS* and *ARID1A* mutations. These findings, particularly in tumors with poor prognostic histologies, offer opportunities to design clinical trials targeting these molecular pathways.

Several different strategies have been advocated for targeted approaches to ovarian cancer, generally involving identification of a gene or protein that is overexpressed and can be reasonably targeted with acceptable toxicity (Figure 8.2). Clinically relevant approaches,

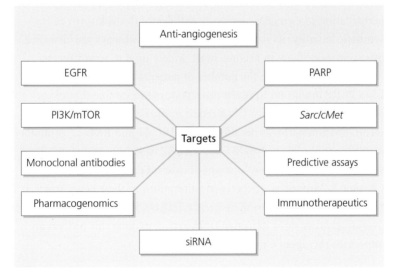

Figure 8.2 Potential approaches to personalized medicine in ovarian cancer. EGFR, epidermal growth factor receptor; mTOR, molecular target of rapamycin; PARP, poly (ADP-ribose) polymerase; PI3K, phosphoinositide 3-kinase; siRNA: small interfering RNA.

or those that are likely to become so in the near future, are discussed in this chapter.

PARP inhibition

Mechanism of action. Poly (ADP-ribose) polymerase (PARP) is a key enzyme involved in the repair of DNA single-strand breaks. If the breaks are not repaired, they accumulate, which in turn results in double-strand breaks leading to cell death. Double-strand breaks are repaired via a high-fidelity repair system known as homologous recombination; the BRCA protein plays a key role in this process, hence intact *BRCA1* and *BRCA2* function is essential for homologous recombination.

Inhibition of the PARP pathway in the presence of *BRCA1* or *BRCA2* mutations means that DNA repair occurs via pathways that lack high fidelity. This can result in multiple replication errors leading to chromosomal instability and apoptotic cell death (Figure 8.3). The inter-relationship between PARP inhibitors and *BRCA* mutations offers a novel therapeutic strategy, whereby the simultaneous perturbation of two genes results in cell death: this is known as synthetic lethality. As more critical genes and pathways are identified, this strategy is likely to become more widely used to treat cancers.

Strategies to increase the number of patients who would benefit from PARP inhibition have led investigators to examine the role of other genes that influence DNA repair in the homologous recombination pathway. In addition to *BRCA1* and *BRCA2*, a number of other genes such as *RAD51* and *PALB2* have been shown to play a significant role in the development of ovarian cancer, as described in Chapter 3. Mutations or epigenetic alterations in these genes result in homologous recombination deficiency (HRD). Up to 50% of epithelial ovarian cancers show defective DNA repair, making this process an important therapeutic target.

PARP inhibitors. Four PARP inhibitors have been developed for use in ovarian cancer: olaparib, rucaparib, niraparib and veliparib. They appear to have similar efficacy, although further data are needed to confirm this initial impression. Preclinical data have shown some

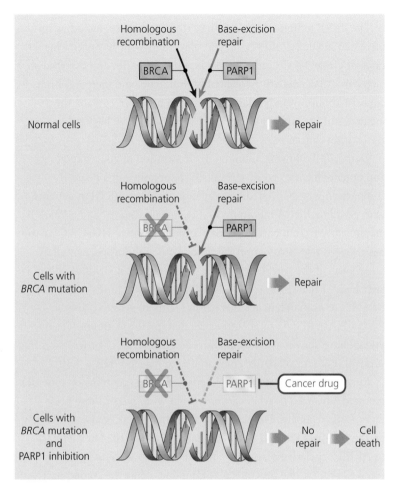

Figure 8.3 DNA strand breaks are usually repaired by the base excision repair mechanism via the enzyme poly (ADP-ribose) polymerase (PARP) and through the homologous recombination mechanism in which the BRCA protein plays a key role. If a cell inherits a *BRCA* mutation, it will only be able to initiate repair via the base excision repair/PARP pathway. However, if a PARP inhibitor is administered, the PARP/base excision repair mechanism is no longer viable either and the DNA cannot be repaired, which leads to cell death.

differences such as the higher tumor penetration observed with niraparib versus olaparib,[2] but the clinical implications of these data remain unclear.

The PARP inhibitors have distinct toxicity profiles, including an increased incidence of liver enzyme elevations with rucaparib, higher rates of grade 3/4 thrombocytopenia with niraparib, and diarrhea with olaparib. All agents are associated with fatigue, and there has been concern about myelodysplastic syndrome; however, to date, the incidence of the latter does not appear to exceed the background rate for ovarian cancer.

Olaparib. Following an initial demonstration of good tolerability and potent efficacy,[3] positive results were obtained in a Phase II comparison with pegylated liposomal doxorubicin (PLD) in patients with germline *BRCA* mutations and recurrent disease,[4] and a Phase II maintenance trial in patients with platinum-sensitive HGSC.[5] Olaparib has received regulatory approval in the USA and Europe, as well as other parts of the world: depending on the region, it is indicated for later lines of therapy in patients with germline mutations in *BRCA1* or *BRCA2*, or as maintenance therapy in platinum-sensitive disease. Recent Phase III data on maintenance therapy for platinum-sensitive disease have shown a significant advantage in terms of progression-free survival (PFS) for olaparib, compared with placebo (HR = 0.30).[6]

Rucaparib is indicated for deleterious *BRCA* (germline or somatic) mutated advanced ovarian cancer treated with two or more prior therapeutic regimens. Development of rucaparib has been based largely on the two-part Phase II ARIEL2 trial[7] and Study 10. The first part of ARIEL2 included platinum-sensitive patients who had previously received at least one previous platinum line, while the second part included those with three or four lines of treatment, including both platinum-sensitive and platinum-resistant disease. In Part 1 of this study, PFS was longer in patients with *BRCA* mutant or *BRCA* wild-type and loss of heterozygosity (LOH) high platinum-sensitive ovarian carcinomas than in those with *BRCA* wild-type LOH low carcinomas.[7]

Niraparib has been evaluated in the Phase III NOVA trial in two cohorts of patients with or without germline *BRCA* mutations, who had achieved a complete or partial response to a platinum-containing regimen.[8] Niraparib improved PFS in both cohorts, with an HR of 0.27 in the germline *BRCA* mutation-positive cohort, 0.38 for patients with no germline mutation but with HRD, and 0.45 for all patients with no germline mutation. Thus, there was benefit across all populations regardless of biomarker status. As a result, niraparib has received regulatory approval in the USA for maintenance treatment of all women with recurrent ovarian cancer regardless of biomarker status.

Veliparib is another highly selective PARP inhibitor that has been developed for the treatment of ovarian cancer. The largest trial in ovarian cancer with this compound is currently recruiting participants with newly diagnosed stage III or IV high-grade serous, epithelial ovarian, fallopian tube or primary peritoneal cancer to investigate the role of PARP inhibition with carboplatin and paclitaxel and as front-line continuation maintenance therapy.

Future trends. Current studies are investigating combinations of PARP inhibitors with anti-angiogenic therapies and immuno-oncologics (see below). In addition, most PARP inhibitors are being assessed in earlier lines of therapy, including front-line treatment.

Anti-angiogenesis therapies

Therapies that target angiogenesis and associated growth factors, such as vascular endothelial growth factor (VEGF), platelet-derived growth factor (PDGF) and fibroblast growth factor (FGF), have been shown to inhibit new blood vessel growth, which in turn leads to tumor regression. There are a number of angiogenesis pathways that represent promising therapeutic targets; indeed, to date, inhibition of angiogenesis has been the most successful targeted strategy in ovarian cancer.

Bevacizumab, a monoclonal antibody directed against VEGF, has been the most widely studied anti-angiogenic agent in ovarian cancer. Initial single-agent activity has been demonstrated in recurrent ovarian cancer in both platinum-sensitive and -resistant disease: Table 8.1 details the various trials by line of therapy. In addition, results from the ENGOT-ov15/AGO OVAR 17 study are pending.[9] However, regulatory approval has lacked harmonization globally: some countries have limited approval to use in recurrent disease, whereas others have permitted use in front-line treatment. Major adverse effects of bevacizumab include hypertension, proteinuria, gastrointestinal perforation or fistula and thromboembolic disease.

TABLE 8.1

Clinical trials with bevacizumab in ovarian cancer

Study	Patients	Treatment
Front-line treatment		
GOG218[10]	Patients with newly diagnosed stage III / IV disease (incompletely or completely debulked) (n = 1873)	*All patients*: Carboplatin (AUC 6 mg/mL/min) + paclitaxel, 175 mg/m² (cycles 1–6) Study treatments (cycles 2–22): BV, 15 mg/kg throughout (BV-throughout) BV, 15 mg/kg (cycles 2–6), Placebo (cycles 7–22) (BV-initiation) Placebo (control) All cycles were 21 days
ICON7[11]	Patients with stage I/IIA (grade 3, clear cell) disease or stage IIB–IV disease (n = 1528)	Carboplatin (AUC 5–6 mg/mL/min) + paclitaxel, 175 mg/m² every 3 weeks Carboplatin (AUC 5–6 mg/mL/min) + paclitaxel, 175 mg/m² + BV, 7.5 mg/kg every 3 weeks Treatment continued for up to 24 cycles or until disease progression
GOG252[12]	Patients with stage II–III disease, resected to optimal (≤ 1 cm visible tumor) (n = 1560)	*Cycles 1–6*: Carboplatin (AUC 6 mg/mL/min) IV + paclitaxel, 80 mg/m² IV over 1 hour + BV, 15 mg/kg IV Carboplatin (AUC 6 mg/mL/min) IP + paclitaxel, 80 mg/m² IV over 1 hour + BV, 15 mg/kg IV Cisplatin 75 mg/m² + paclitaxel, 135 mg/m² IV over 3 hours on day 1 and 60 mg/m² IP on day 8 + BV, 15 mg/kg IV *Cycles 7–22*: BV, 15 mg/kg IV on day 1

Principal comparisons	Primary endpoint	Key results PFS	OS
Short- or long-term BV vs control	PFS	*Control*: median 10.3 months	*Control:* median 39.3 months
		BV-throughout: median 14.1 months (HR 0.72, $p < 0.001$)	*BV-throughout*: median 39.7 months (HR 0.89)
		BV-initiation: median 11.2 months (HR 0.91, $p = 0.16$)	*BV-initiation*: median 38.7 months (HR 1.08)
BV + CT vs CT alone	PFS, OS	*Control*: median 17.4 months	*Control*: median not reached
		BV: 19.8 months (HR 0.87, $p = 0.04$)	*BV*: median not reached (HR 0.85, $p = 0.11$)
IP carboplatin vs IV carboplatin	PFS	*IV carboplatin:* median 26.8 months	Results pending
		IP carboplatin: median 28.7 months (HR 0.95, $p = 0.416$)	
		IP cisplatin: median 27.8 months (HR 1.01, $p = 0.727$)	

CONTINUED

TABLE 8.1 (CONTINUED)

Clinical trials with bevacizumab in ovarian cancer

Study	Patients	Treatment

Recurrent disease

Study	Patients	Treatment
GOG213[13]	Patients with platinum-sensitive recurrent disease, who were candidates for cytoreduction surgery (n = 674)	Patients eligible for surgery underwent cytoreduction, followed by randomization to CT arms. Patients who were ineligible for surgery could receive CT after randomization. *CT regimens:* Carboplatin (AUC 5 mg/mL/min) + paclitaxel, 175 mg/m² Carboplatin (AUC 5 mg/mL/min) + paclitaxel, 175 mg/m² + BV 15 mg/kg
AURELIA[14]	Patients with platinum-resistant recurrent epithelial ovarian cancer who received ≤ 2 previous lines of therapy; no rectosigmoidal involvement (n = 361)	CT (investigator's choice of: PLD, 40 mg/m²; topotecan, 4 mg/m² weekly or 1.25 mg/m² on days 1–5; or paclitaxel, 80 mg/m² weekly) CT + BV, 10 mg/kg every 2 weeks or every 3 weeks if given with topotecan Treatment continued to disease progression, unacceptable toxicity or withdrawal of consent
OCEANS[15]	Patients with platinum-sensitive disease with recurrence ≥ 6 months after first-line platinum-based therapy (n = 484)	Carboplatin (AUC 4 mg/mL/min) + gemcitabine, 1000 mg/m² Carboplatin (AUC 4 mg/mL/min) + gemcitabine, 1000 mg/m² + BV, 15 mg/kg Treatment continued for 6–10 cycles

AUC, area under the (concentration vs time) curve; BV, bevacizumab; CT, chemotherapy; IP, intraperitoneal; IV, intravenous; OS, overall survival; PFS, progression-free survival.

Principal comparisons	Primary endpoint	Key results	
		PFS	OS
BV + CT vs CT alone	OS	Control: median 10.4 months	Control: median 37.3 months
Cytoreduction vs no cytoreduction		BV: median 13.8 months (HR 0.61, $p < 0.0001$)	BV: median 42.6 months (HR 0.84, $p = 0.056$)
		Results for cytoreduction vs no cytoreduction comparison is pending	Results for cytoreduction vs no cytoreduction comparison is pending
BV + CT vs CT alone	PFS	CT alone: median 3.4 months	CT alone: median 13.3 months
		BV: median 6.7 months (HR 0.48, $p \leq 0.0001$)	BV: median 16.6 months (HR 0.85, $p = 0.174$)
BV + CT vs CT alone	PFS	Control: 8.4 months	Control: median 35.2 months
		BV: median 12.4 months (HR 0.48, $p < 0.0001$)	BV: median 33.3 months
			Data remain immature

Note: other anti-angiogenic agents have been studied in ovarian cancer, including cediranib, pazopanib, nintedanib and trebananib. These agents are less specific as they target multiple pathways that include vascular endothelial growth factor (VEGF), fibroblast growth factor (FGF), platelet-derived growth factor (PDGF) and angiopoietin.

Immuno-oncologics

Interest in manipulating the immune system to combat cancers has expanded dramatically in recent years. The concept is that if the immune system can learn to recognize malignant cells as foreign antigens, a robust T-cell mediated response, among other pathways, could be induced. Cancer cells evade these tumor-directed T cells by subverting immune checkpoint pathways and other immune-regulatory mechanisms. This observation has led to the identification of numerous targets and therapeutic strategies with checkpoint inhibitors and other agents (Figure 8.4). Checkpoint proteins, such as programmed cell death (PD)-1, prevent the immune system from activating a response, and some tumor cells are able to express the ligand that binds to this protein (PD-L1), thereby suppressing an immune response. Antibodies that target the PD-1 protein or its ligand can block this suppression and thereby activate an immune response.

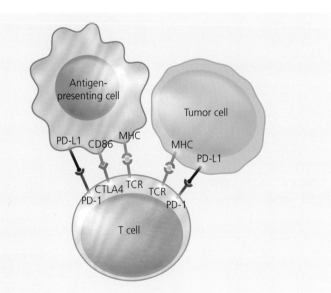

Figure 8.4 Potential immuno-oncologic targets in ovarian cancer. CD86, cluster of differentiation 86; CTLA4, cytotoxic T-lymphocyte-associated protein 4; MHC, major histocompatibility complex; PD-1, programmed cell death protein 1; PD-L1, programmed cell death ligand 1; TCR, T-cell receptor. Adapted from Gaillard SL et al. 2016.[16]

Another important protein on the T cell, which if bound and activated can suppress an immune response, is cytotoxic T-lymphocyte-associated protein 4 (CTLA-4).

Table 8.2 shows examples of some of the principal compounds currently under investigation in ovarian cancer. These agents have shown remarkable long-term responses in multiple solid tumors, and are approved in a number of cancers including melanoma, non-small-

TABLE 8.2

Immuno-oncologic therapies currently under investigation in ovarian cancer[16]

Drug	Target	Type of antibody	Current approved indications (Europe/FDA)
Nivolumab	PD-1	Fully humanized IgG4	Melanoma NSCLC Renal cell carcinoma Hodgkin's lymphoma
Pembrolizumab	PD-1	Humanized IgG4	Melanoma NSCLC
Ipilimumab	CTLA-4	Recombinant human IgG1	Melanoma
Atezolizumab	PD-L1	Fc-engineered, humanized, non-glycosylated IgG1-κ	Urothelial/bladder carcinoma (FDA only)
Avelumab	PD-L1	Fully humanized IgG1	In development
Durvalumab	PD-L1	Fc-optimized IgG1	FDA breakthrough designation for PD-L1-positive urothelial bladder cancer

CTLA-4, cytotoxic T-lymphocyte-associated protein 4; Fc, fragment crystallizable (region); FDA, Food and Drug Administration (USA); Ig, immunoglobulin; NSCLC, non-small-cell lung cancer; PD-1, programmed cell death protein 1; PD-L1, programmed cell death ligand 1.

cell lung cancer, renal cancer, bladder cancer, head and neck cancer and urothelial cancers. Given their mechanisms of action, these agents may show survival benefit without inducing a significant objective response. Thus, alternative assessment criteria using an immune derivation of the conventional clinical Response Evaluation Criteria In Solid Tumors (RECIST) has been developed.[17] It should be noted that these agents can cause significant and life-threatening adverse effects, including inflammation of the liver, lungs and colon.

It has been suggested that a combination of immune agents with PARP inhibitors might be beneficial, because tumor mutations and DNA alterations can generate neo-antigens that have been associated with an improved response to immune checkpoint therapies. Preclinical data suggest that exposure to PARP inhibitors increases the neo-antigen load, thereby making immunotherapeutic agents more effective. Clinical trials are in development to investigate this theory.[16]

Key points – targeted therapies

- Precision medicine has become a key strategy in ovarian cancer.
- There is great hope that targeted therapies will offer improved outcomes.
- Targeted therapy generally involves identifying a gene or protein that is overexpressed in cancer and can be reasonably targeted with acceptable toxicity.
- Poly (ADP-ribose) polymerase (PARP) inhibitors– olaparib, rucaparib, niraparib and veliparib – appear to be comparable in efficacy, but have differing toxicity profiles.
- Inhibition of tumor angiogenesis is the most successful targeted therapy strategy in ovarian cancer.
- Bevacizumab has shown activity as a single agent in recurrent ovarian cancer in both platinum-sensitive and -resistant disease.
- A number of immuno-oncologic therapies, including inhibitors of programmed cell death protein 1 (PD-1) and its ligand (PD-L1), have shown efficacy in various solid tumors and are under active development in ovarian cancer.

References

1 McCluggage WG. My approach to and thoughts on the typing of ovarian carcinomas. *J Clin Pathol* 2008;61:152–63.

2 Mikule K, Wang S, Weroha SJ et al. A preclinical evaluation of niraparib efficacy as monotherapy, maintenance and after olaparib treatment (PARP inhibitor after PARP inhibitor) in patient-derived ovarian xenograft tumor models. *Eur J Cancer* 2017;72(Suppl 1):S96.

3 Fong PC, Boss DS, Yap TA et al. Inhibition of poly(ADP-ribose) polymerase in tumors from BRCA mutation carriers. *N Engl J Med* 2009;361:123–34.

4 Kaye SB, Lubinski J, Matulonis U et al. Phase II, open-label, randomized, multicenter study comparing the efficacy and safety of olaparib, a poly (ADP-ribose) polymerase inhibitor, and pegylated liposomal doxorubicin in patients with BRCA1 or BRCA2 mutations and recurrent ovarian cancer. *J Clin Oncol* 2012;30:372–9.

5 Ledermann J, Harter P, Gourley C et al. Olaparib maintenance therapy in platinum-sensitive relapsed ovarian cancer. *N Engl J Med* 2012;366:1382–92.

6 Pujade-Lauraine JA, Ledermann RT, Penson AM et al. Treatment with olaparib monotherapy in the maintenance setting significantly improves progression-free survival in patients with platinum-sensitive relapsed ovarian cancer: results from the phase III SOLO2 study. Presented at the Society of Gynecologic Oncology, National Harbor, MD, 12–15 March 2017.

7 Swisher EM, Lin KK, Oza AM et al. Rucaparib in relapsed, platinum-sensitive high-grade ovarian carcinoma (ARIEL2 Part 1): an international, multicentre, open-label, phase 2 trial. *Lancet Oncol* 2017;18:75–87.

8 Mirza MR, Monk BJ, Herrstedt J et al. Niraparib maintenance therapy in platinum-sensitive, recurrent ovarian cancer. *N Engl J Med* 2016;375:2154–64.

9 www.clinicaltrialsregister.eu/ctr-search/trial/2011–001015–32/FR, last accessed 09 March 2017.

10 Burger RA, Brady MF, Bookman MA et al.; Gynecologic Oncology Group. Incorporation of bevacizumab in the primary treatment of ovarian cancer. *N Engl J Med* 2011;365:2473–83.

11 Perren TJ, Swart AM, Pfisterer J et al.; ICON7 investigators. A phase 3 trial of bevacizumab in ovarian cancer. *N Engl J Med* 2011;365:2484–96.

12 Walker JL, Brady MF, DiSilvestro PA et al. A Phase III clinical trial of bevacizumab with iv versus ip chemotherapy in ovarian, fallopian tube and primary peritoneal carcinoma nci-supplied agent(s): bevacizumab (NSC #704865, IND #7921) NCT01167712 a GOG/NRG trial (GOG 252). Presented at the Society of Gynecologic Oncology's Annual Meeting on Women's Cancer, 19–22 March 2016, San Diego, California, USA.

13 Coleman RL, Brady RF, Herzog TJ et al. A phase III randomized controlled clinical trial of carboplatin and paclitaxel alone or in combination with bevacizumab followed by bevacizumab and secondary cytoreductive surgery in platinum-sensitive, recurrent ovarian, peritoneal primary and fallopian tube cancer. Presented at Society of Gynecologic Oncology's Annual Meeting on Women's Cancer 2015, 28–31 March 2015, Chicago, Illinois, USA. Abstract 3. www.roche.com/dam/jcr:3050d757–8d1d–48a6-b372-c72dc3715556/en/med-cor–2016–12–07-e.pdf and http://www.onclive.com/conference-coverage/sgo–2015/bevacizumab-regimen-extends-survival-in-phase-iii-ovarian-cancer-trial (both accessed 09 March 2017).

14 Pujade-Lauraine E, Hilpert F, Weber B et al. Bevacizumab combined with chemotherapy for platinum-resistant recurrent ovarian cancer: the AURELIA open-label randomized phase III trial. *J Clin Oncol* 2014;32:1302–8.

15 Aghajanian C, Blank SV, Goff BA et al. OCEANS: a randomized, double-blind, placebo-controlled phase III trial of chemotherapy with or without bevacizumab in patients with platinum-sensitive recurrent epithelial ovarian, primary peritoneal, or fallopian tube cancer. *J Clin Oncol* 2012;30:2039–45.

16 Gaillard SL, Secord AA, Monk B. The role of immune checkpoint inhibition in the treatment of ovarian cancer. *Gynecol Oncol Res Pract* 2016;3:11.

17 Seymour L, Bogaerts J, Perrone A et al. iRECIST: guidelines for response criteria for use in trials testing immunotherapeutics. *Lancet Oncol* 2017;18:e143–52.

Further reading

Jackson AL, Davenport SM, Herzog TJ, Coleman RL. Targeting angiogenesis: vascular endothelial growth factor and related signaling pathways. *Transl Cancer Res* 2015;4:70–83.

Non-epithelial tumors are rare, accounting for 10–15% of all ovarian malignant neoplasms.[1,2] The most common types are germ cell tumors (GCTs) and sex cord–stromal tumors (SCSTs) (Table 9.1). The prognosis of non-epithelial ovarian neoplasms tends to be better than for epithelial cancers, largely because most tend to present at an earlier stage: 60–70% of GCTs and 60–95% of SCSTs are detected at an early stage.[1,2] They will commonly present at younger ages, compared with the more common epithelial ovarian cancer.

Germ cell tumors

Malignant germ cell tumors arising in the ovary (MOGCT) are estimated to affect about 60 women each year in England. They typically occur in older adolescents and young women, but rarely may also occur in the postmenopausal population. In most instances, no predisposing factors are found. In rare cases, these tumors can arise from fully differentiated teratomas or dermoids, which are more common and benign conditions. In addition, several very rare syndromes linked with gonadal dysgenesis, including Turner and Swyer syndrome, have been associated with MOGCT, and it remains possible that there could be exceptionally rare families with increased risk, as seen in malignant testicular germ cell tumors.

Since germ cells can differentiate to form all cell types seen in neonates and adults, any combination of pathologies is possible, although some are more common than others. For example, elements of yolk sac tumor, choriocarcinoma and dysgerminoma are more commonly seen than embryonal or rhabdomyosarcoma. The elements present can help to predict clinical behavior and the production of tumor markers.

Tumor markers. Patients with choriocarcinoma/trophoblastic tumor elements will usually have elevated serum human chorionic gonadotropin (hCG), and those with yolk sac tumors will produce

TABLE 9.1

Classification of the most common non-epithelial ovarian cancers[1]

Germ cell tumors

- Dysgerminoma
- Yolk sac (endodermal sinus) tumors
- Embryonal carcinoma
- Polyembryoma
- Choriocarcinoma
- Teratoma
  - immature teratoma
  - mature teratoma

Mixed type (≥ 2 of the above types)

Sex cord–stromal tumors

- Granulosa cell tumors
  - adult type
  - juvenile type
- Theca–fibroma group
  - thecoma
  - fibroma
  - fibrosarcoma
  - sclerosing stromal tumor
  - signet-ring stromal tumor
- Sertoli–stromal tumor
  - well differentiated
  - intermediate differentiation
  - poorly differentiated
  - retiform
- SCST of mixed or unclassified cell type
  - gynandroblastoma
  - SCST, unclassified

Metastatic tumors

SCST, sex cord–stromal tumor.

alpha-fetoprotein (AFP) (Table 9.2). Elevation of either or both of these two markers is seen in about 85% of non-dysgerminomatous MOGCT, and hCG is also raised in about 10% of dysgerminomatous cases. In addition, CA125 may be non-specifically raised in any type of MOGCT induced by peritoneal irritation. Thus, measurement of AFP, hCG and CA125 can help in the diagnostic work-up of patients with a suspected ovarian mass, and should be done in any woman under the age of 50 years who wants a fertility-sparing approach to treatment. This is because elevated hCG or AFP is virtually diagnostic of MOGCT, and could lead to fertility-sparing surgery rather than the usual more radical surgery used for primary epithelial cancers.

Clinical presentation and investigations. Usually patients present with only a short history of lower abdominal swelling and pain arising from the pelvis, as these tumors tend to grow rapidly. Local and/or systemic impairment and pain can arise in combination with an irregular menstrual cycle.

TABLE 9.2

Serum tumor markers in malignant germ cell tumors of the ovary

Histology	AFP	hCG
Dysgerminoma	–	+
Immature teratoma	+	–
Yolk sac tumor	+	–
Choriocarcinoma	–	+
Embryonal carcinoma	+	+
Polyembryoma	±	+
Mixed GCT	±	±

AFP, alpha-fetoprotein; GCT, germ cell tumor; hCG, human chorionic gonadotropin.

Sex cord–stromal tumors

SCSTs arise from the sex cords and ovarian stroma, and account for 5–8% of ovarian cancers.[1] The diagnosis of an SCST should be suspected in patients with:

- an adnexal mass on ultrasound
- estrogen excess with precocious puberty
- abnormal uterine bleeding
- endometrial hyperplasia
- androgen excess with virilization.

Potential biomarkers of SCSTs are shown in Table 9.3.

Granulosa cell tumors are the most common form of SCST, and account for 2–5% of all ovarian malignant neoplasms.[1] There are two subtypes of granulosa cell tumors: juvenile and adult.

- Juvenile-type tumors account for only 5% of granulosa cell tumors, and typically occur in children and young adults. Histologically, these tumors are characterized by lobulated cells with signs of luteinization.[1]
- Adult-type tumors typically present during the perimenopausal or menopausal period. In this subtype, granulosa cells are arranged in small clusters or rosettes around a central cavity (Call–Exner bodies).

TABLE 9.3

Potential tumor biomarkers secreted by sex cord–stromal tumors of the ovary

Tumor type	Estradiol	Inhibin	T	AE	DHEA
Granulosa cell	+	+	–	–	–
Sertoli–Leydig	–	±	+	+	–
Thecoma–fibroma	–	–	–	–	–
Gonadoblastoma	±	+	±	±	±

AE, androstenedione; DHEA, dehydroepiandrosterone; T, testosterone.

Adult subtype granulosa cell tumors have a microfollicular pattern, while juvenile subtypes present with a macrofollicular or cystic pattern. The nuclei are often described as coffee bean-like in morphology.

Treatment. Unilateral salpingo-oophorectomy (see Figure 5.1, page 41) with adequate peritoneal staging should be considered as a fertility-preserving option for patients with stage I disease. If the uterus is preserved, an evaluation of the endometrium, for example through dilatation and curettage, should be performed to exclude an estrogen-induced endometrial cancerous or precancerous state. Systematic lymph node dissection or sampling has no value in the absence of bulky nodes. Similarly, there is no value in blind biopsies of a normal contralateral ovary.

Maximal effort debulking surgery, aiming at complete cytoreduction, is the most effective treatment for patients with metastatic or recurrent granulosa cell tumors.[2,3] There are no data to support a survival benefit with postoperative chemotherapy for women with resected disease. However, the BEP regimen (bleomycin, etoposide, cisplatin) is usually recommended for women with advanced disease, although the less toxic carboplatin and paclitaxel combination is increasingly being used. In patients with hormone receptor-positive disease, antihormonal treatment has also been shown to be effective.[4]

Sertoli–Leydig cell tumors typically occur during the third and fourth decades of life: about 75% of patients are under 40 years old at diagnosis.[1] They secrete androgens, hence 75–80% of patients show signs of virilization.[1] Typically, patients present with abdominal pain and a palpable abdominal mass.

Treatment. Surgery forms the mainstay of treatment of Sertoli–Leydig cell tumors. Surgical treatment guidelines are similar to those for granulosa cell tumors, with fertility-sparing approaches being considered in early disease and young patients wishing to have children.[1] Platinum-based adjuvant chemotherapy, for example with BEP, is recommended for patients with unresectable or disseminated disease.[2]

Key points – non-epithelial ovarian tumors

- Non-epithelial malignant neoplasms account for 10–15% of ovarian cancers.
- They occur at younger ages than the more common epithelial ovarian cancer.
- Adequate surgical staging is essential, and should be performed even when fertility-sparing surgery is planned.
- Complete cytoreduction is the cornerstone of treatment in advanced and relapsed disease.
- There is inconclusive evidence for the use of systemic chemotherapy, rather than antihormonal treatment, in malignant non-epithelial ovarian tumors. In completely resected disease, there is little evidence to support a survival benefit with additional systemic treatment.

References

1 Boussios S, Zarkavelis G, Seraj E et al. Non-epithelial ovarian cancer: elucidating uncommon gynaecological malignancies. *Anticancer Res* 2016;36:5031–42.

2 Colombo N, Peiretti M, Castiglione M; ESMO Guidelines Working Group. Non-epithelial ovarian cancer: ESMO clinical recommendations for diagnosis, treatment and follow-up. *Ann Oncol* 2009;20(Suppl 4):24–6.

3 Fotopoulou C, Savvatis K, Braicu EI et al. Adult granulosa cell tumors of the ovary: tumor dissemination pattern at primary and recurrent situation, surgical outcome. *Gynecol Oncol* 2010;119:285–90.

4 Colombo N, Parma G, Zanagnolo V, Insinga A. Management of ovarian stromal cell tumors. *J Clin Oncol* 2007;25:2944–51.

Further reading

Ray-Coquard I, Weber B, Lotz JP et al. Management of rare ovarian cancers: the experience of the French website "Observatory for rare malignant tumors of the ovaries" by the GINECO group: interim analysis of the first 100 patients. *Gynecol Oncol* 2010;119:53–9.

Witkowski L, McCluggage WG, Foulkes WD. Recently characterized molecular events in uncommon gynaecological neoplasms and their clinical importance. *Histopathology* 2016;69:903–13.

As in all cancer care, the follow-up of patients with ovarian cancer mostly lacks any prospective randomized evidence basis: guidelines are largely based on tradition, the wishes and experiences of patients and physicians, and rather arbitrary timelines depending on the type of examinations performed. In general, follow-up aims not only to diagnose relapse, but also to holistically assess and manage ongoing physical, psychological, emotional, financial and sexual survivorship issues.

Nevertheless, to date, no prospective evidence has shown that such follow-up results in a significant survival benefit in patients with ovarian cancer.

Follow-up

Traditionally, in accordance with various national and international guidelines, patients are followed up at 3-month intervals in the first 3 years, and 6-month intervals thereafter, depending on their symptoms and overall clinical picture. However, follow-up practice varies markedly, and each center usually has its own guidelines and protocols, without any evidence for the superiority of one approach over another. Typically, follow-up consists of an interview with the patient, assessment of any potential tumor-related symptoms, clinical examination and possibly also investigations for the diagnosis of common tumor-related symptoms (Table 10.1).

Serial measurement of CA125 often forms part of follow-up, because elevations of CA125 precede symptomatic relapse by a median of 4.5 months (range 0.5–29.5 months). However, this approach failed to demonstrate any significant effect on patients' survival in the UK-based prospective randomized MRC/EORTC trial, in which there was no difference in overall survival between patients who received chemotherapy based on a rising CA125 level and those who did not receive chemotherapy until they were symptomatic (Figure 10.1).[1] In this study, however, only 6% of the patients

TABLE 10.1

Typical follow-up of ovarian cancer patients*

- Patient interview
- Assessment of tumor-related symptoms (pain etc.)
- Clinical evaluation
- Transvaginal/transabdominal ultrasound for diagnosis of tumor-related symptoms (ascites, pleural effusion, hydronephrosis etc.)

*Practice patterns vary between countries and centers.

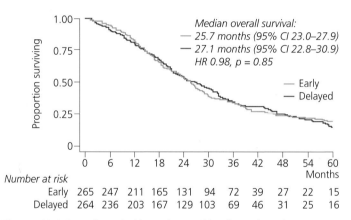

Median overall survival:
— 25.7 months (95% CI 23.0–27.9)
— 27.1 months (95% CI 22.8–30.9)
HR 0.98, p = 0.85

Number at risk	0	6	12	18	24	30	36	42	48	54	60
Early	265	247	211	165	131	94	72	39	27	22	15
Delayed	264	236	203	167	129	103	69	46	31	25	16

Figure 10.1 Overall survival in patients with relapsed ovarian cancer according to timing of chemotherapy (early versus delayed). Reproduced with permission from Rustin GJ et al 2010.[1]

underwent surgery for relapsed disease. Depending on the final analysis of the DESKTOP III survival data, follow-up for ovarian cancer may need to be reshaped and redefined, as it may be worthwhile detecting the disease while it is apparently operable and when the patient has a good performance status.

The emerging trend of targeted maintenance treatments for advanced ovarian cancer is also reshaping the approach to follow-up, since in this situation patients are visiting their oncologists over prolonged periods, and assessments of treatment efficacy and adverse events are performed regularly.

Patients undergoing fertility-sparing treatment should receive regular ultrasonographic examination of the contralateral ovary and the endometrial cavity to diagnose relapse in the remaining Müllerian organs. Depending on the initial stage, the patient's wishes and reproductive history and her overall response to cancer treatment, removal of the uterus and contralateral ovary may be discussed after completion of childbearing.

There is increasing interest in the impact of psycho-oncologic support interventions in women treated for ovarian cancer. Numerous studies are addressing the potential long-term effect of such interventions.

Palliative salvage surgery

Patients with epithelial ovarian cancer often present with symptoms of impaired intestinal transit or clinical bowel obstruction at relapse, which is attributable to the diffuse peritoneal dissemination of recurrent tumor. The use of novel targeted therapies with anti-angiogenic potential may favor fistula formation or intestinal perforation, and so recurrent epithelial ovarian cancer with the potential for such severe acute complications constitutes a therapeutic dilemma.[2] Palliative surgery in patients with gastrointestinal and other symptoms of ovarian cancer recurrence therefore requires a multidisciplinary approach.[3]

Risks versus benefits. Any perceived benefits should be carefully balanced against the risks for each individual patient along with factors such as comorbidities, baseline quality of life, previous response to chemotherapy, length of treatment intervals and the patient's wishes. The management of these cases should be led by specialist gynecologic multidisciplinary teams. Intraoperative input from gynecologic oncologists is important to ensure that both the meaningful responses possible after palliative surgery and the likelihood of disease response to chemotherapy are duly considered when making intraoperative decisions.

Endoscopic techniques such as placement of intestinal stents and percutaneous endoscopic gastrostomy (PEG) may allow the palliation

95

of gastrointestinal symptoms, with reduced procedure-related morbidity in selected patients. Surgical intervention should be restricted to patients who have a distal mechanical bowel obstruction and in whom the formation of a proximal small bowel stoma is not likely to be necessary, as such high-output stomas significantly reduce patients' quality of life and necessitate permanent total parenteral nutrition.

Preoperative imaging demonstrating the most proximal point of bowel obstruction should be used to identify patients with a level of obstruction that presents a high risk of iatrogenic short bowel syndrome. The severe peritoneal carcinomatosis and inflammation present in epithelial ovarian cancer recurrence makes surgical dissection hazardous, and renders the successful repair of enterotomies without fistula formation challenging. Considering the balance of risk and benefits, few patients are suitable for palliative defunctioning or bypass procedures, and therefore multidisciplinary teams with experience in managing such cases and their potential complications should be responsible for the careful selection and care of those who do undergo surgery.[4]

Key points – follow-up and palliative surgery

- The value, type and role of follow-up in cancer care is not well defined and prospective randomized trials are scarce.
- The type of follow-up depends on whether the patient has undergone fertility-sparing surgery.
- Serial CA125 measurements have failed to show any survival benefit over observation alone.
- Follow-up should involve holistic aspects and psycho-oncologic support.
- Palliative surgery should be performed only after all conservative management options have been exhausted.
- Short bowel syndrome is a common complication after palliative surgery for bowel obstruction in relapsed disease.

References

1 Rustin GJ, van der Burg ME, Griffin CL et al. Early versus delayed treatment of relapsed ovarian cancer (MRC OV05/EORTC 55955): a randomised trial. *Lancet* 2010;376:1155–63.

2 Burger RA, Brady MF, Bookman MA et al. Risk factors for GI adverse events in a phase III randomized trial of bevacizumab in first-line therapy of advanced ovarian cancer: a Gynecologic Oncology Group Study. *J Clin Oncol* 2014;32:1210–17.

3 Fotopoulou C, Zang R, Gultekin M et al. Value of tertiary cytoreductive surgery in epithelial ovarian cancer: an international multicenter evaluation. *Ann Surg Oncol* 2013;20:1348–54.

4 Fotopoulou C, Braicu EI, Kwee SL et al. Salvage surgery due to bowel obstruction in advanced or relapsed ovarian cancer resulting in short bowel syndrome and long-life total parenteral nutrition: surgical and clinical outcome. *Int J Gynecol Cancer* 2013;23:1495–500.

Useful resources

UK
Cancer Research UK
Speak to a Nurse: 0808 800 4040
Tel: 0300 123 1022
www.cancerresearchuk.org

Macmillan Cancer Support
CancerLine: 0808 808 00 00
www.macmillan.org.uk

Marie Curie Cancer Care
Support Line: 0800 090 2309
Health professionals: 0845 056
7899
www.mariecurie.org.uk

Ovarian Cancer Action
Tel: +44 (0)20 7380 1730
www.ovarian.org.uk

USA
American Cancer Society
Helpline: +1 800 227 2345
www.cancer.org

American Congress of
Obstetricians and Gynecologists
Toll-free: 1 800 673 8444
Tel: +1 202 638 5577
www.acog.org

Cancercare
Tel: +1 800 813 4673
www.cancercare.org

Foundation for Women's Cancer
Tel: +1 312 578 1439
www.foundationforwomenscancer.org

HERA Women's Cancer
Foundation
Tel: +1 970 948 7360
www.herafoundation.org

National Comprehensive Cancer
Network
Tel: +1 215 690 0300
www.nccn.org

National Ovarian Cancer
Coalition
InfoLine: +1 888 682 7426
www.ovarian.org

Ovarian Cancer Awareness
Foundation
Tel: +1 901 373 2372
www.ocafoundation.org

Ovarian Cancer Research Fund
Alliance
Tel: +1 212 268 1002
www.ocrfa.org

SHARE Self-help for women with breast or ovarian cancer
Toll-free: +1 844 275 7427
Tel: +1 212 719 0364
www.sharecancersupport.org

Society of Gynecologic Oncology
Tel:+1 312 235 4060
www.sgo.org

International
Cancer Association of South Africa
Toll-free: 0800 22 6622
www.cansa.org.za

Cancer Australia
Toll-free: 1800 624 973
Tel: +61 (0)2 9357 9400
www.canceraustralia.gov.au

International Federation of Gynecology and Obstetrics (FIGO)
Tel: +44 (0)20 7928 1166
www.figo.org

International Gynecologic Cancer Society
Tel: +1 502 891 4575
www.igcs.org

Ovarian Cancer Australia
Tel: 1300 660 334
www.ovariancancer.net.au

Ovarian Cancer Canada
Toll-free: 1 877 413 7970
Tel: +1 416 962 2700
www.ovariancanada.org

FastTest

You've read the book ... now test yourself with key questions from the authors

- Go to the FastTest for this title *FREE* at fastfacts.com
- Approximate time **10 minutes**
- For best retention of the key issues, try taking the FastTest before and after reading

Index

FF ▶ *Fast Facts*

Reading for results
(and tests worth taking)

With so much to read these days, you need to be selective ...

Was this Fast Facts well worth reading?

Has it helped you make good health decisions?

Did it trigger new ideas you'd like to explore?

If so, please post them in the comments box on the relevant page on **www.fastfacts.com**, and check out fellow readers' insights while you're there.

This is also the place to leave questions for the authors' consideration, and to spend 10 minutes on the free **FastTest** to ensure those key points really sunk in, and that you are set to apply them – **result!**

This Fast Facts has helped me make good health decisions:

| ✔ YES | | **27** |
| ✘ NO | **SUBMIT** ❯ | Good health decisions |

Comments for the authors

Name:

Comment:

Country: Please select ▼

ADD COMMENT ❯

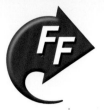
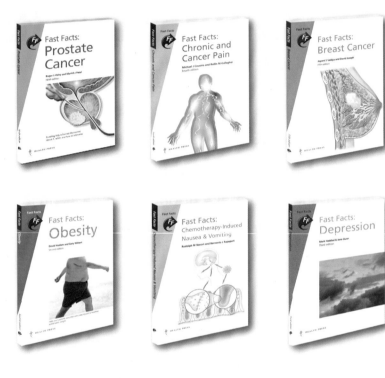
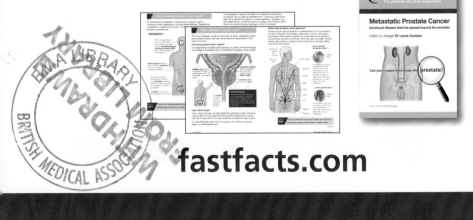